Sam Gueller

THE TOTAL ARTIFICIAL HEART

Past and Future

SynCardia

Compressed Air

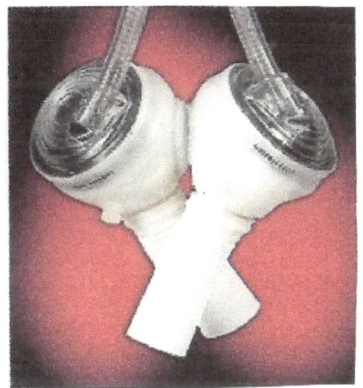

Liotta 1963

Kolff & Jarvik 1992

AbioCor

Electric, Electronic

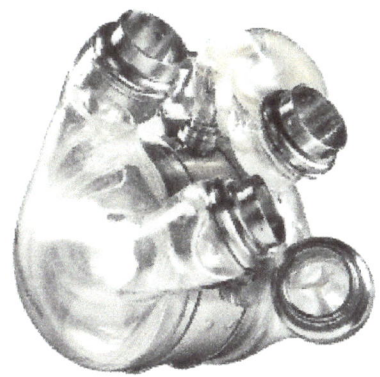

Gueller 1983

Lederman 2001

Other Books by the Author

Fronteras de la Física, Editorial Trazos, Venezuela, 1984

Frontiers of Physics, Vantage Press, New York, 1984

El Origen del Pueblo Judio, Editorial Academica, Madrid, Spain, 2007

Physics Phenomenology, CreateSpace, Charleston SC 2013

Physics of Strings, Second Edition, CreateSpace, Charleston SC 2014

General Math of Nature Phenomena, CreateSpace, Charleston SC 2016

Graphic Art by Artificial Intelligence, CreateSpace, Charleston, SC 2017

ISBN-13: 978-1974062539

ISBN-10: 1974062538

In Memory of Dr. Willem Kolff

Developer of the Artificial Kidney and Pioneer of the Total Artificial Heart

TABLE OF CONTENTS

Introduction	6
The History	7
Accomplishments and Shortcomings	9
Previous Intents	10
Present situation as of Middle 2017	11
The Future	12
Research Design and Methods	12
The Test Bench Method	20
Expcriments with Clinical Implications	26
Guidelines for a 3th Generation of a TAH	30
Annex 1: Figures 1 thru 17 and Forms 1 Thru 6	34
Annex 2 Historic Review	58
Annex 3 Author Credentials	68
Notations	71
Bibliography	72
About the Author	73

INTRODUCTION

The 1960's is the time when the first intent to build a total mechanical heart was made by means of chambers where elastic rubber forced blood to flow under the impulse provided by an external fix compressor's air.

Progress in design, construction and implant followed with increased survival time though was set a goal of 5 years survival but not accomplished, only to several months. In those early years was thought that to pump blood in an electromagnetic field to avoid difficulties was utopic and impossible. The main obstacles for comfort and efficient operation were transcutaneous opening because infection and flow output control to mimic a live total heart, and a compressor at maximum moving on heels and connected to the electric grid. Subsequent advances up to the present increased for and average survival time of 12 months and sometimes a little more with this system.

I suggested in the early 1980 to transfer transcutaneous electric energy without a skin hole to be feed by means of a set of rechargeable belt batteries. The analog pumps themselves were to be driven by a fluid instead of air, these pumps of the positive displacement type. Because electronic was enough advanced at the time, control of pumps rate was included as well as blood flow required data from mayor organs by means of sensors and wiring to a small central processing unit.

In this way, the electric device was borne in concept, in practice an operating one was possible in the middle of 1990 at a great effort and cost. The result was satisfactory with two problems corrected, one was the wiring from the mayor organs which provoked an intolerable discomfort to the patient and was substituted by a colorimetric oxygen detector, and actually an unsurmountable one is the 2 times weight because excessive metal applied, nothing to say of its cost, but remains the most advanced at this writing.

July 2017

THE HISTORY

As time passed, today we observe that the survival time has not increased, even proportionally but remain at about one-year average waiting for a donor transplant. These slow progress is significant if we accept that the original work of the 1960's was a human endeavor trying to build quickly what by nature was developed by millennia, if not millions of years of slow evolution, just because it looked as a pump as seen, really as those used to pump water. In fact, the heart and vascular system doesn't work as a pump in a simple circuit, not pumping an elemental fluid as water. Details of this history can be found in Appendix 2

At present, that is the situation, and after almost more than 50 years it is time to analyze how to proceed further, because one must be indeed. The main obstacles to solve, are to test a total artificial (TAH) in an analog test bench where many runs can be made to get data to improve the design, instead of a shot on a patient whose biological parameters are approximate to said the least.

In the near future research must be focused in those original goals of 5 years survival and electromagnetic pumping a blood flow instead of heavy motors and diaphragms, as well as pump output adjusted to proper patient vascular size and condition.

Here we will outline how it can be accomplished, they are suggestions more than solutions as incentives for a new researches generation, it is all about to revive the spirit of the 1960's for a new push in a convincing thought that it is possible a more perfect TAH that can be built over the years, hoping to be shorter than the one already past.

We will address critical difficulties for additional progress in cardiology and vascular analysis by adding the advantages of simulation techniques to the state of the art of the medical science specific to these fields. The aims of the project will provide an accessible and deeper knowledge of the working system, suggesting the means to deal with, as well as longer lives for patients by itself or by waiting a heart donor. This planning addresses the need to test TAHs before implant, to substitute a human subject, according advanced modeling techniques, which requires the design and construction of a hemodynamic testing bench to be located in a Test Research Station (TRS).

This will be done with the application of dimensional analysis and similitude enabling the organization and simplification of experiments, and in correlation and interpretation of experimental data. Alternative designs of TAHs will be referred to the TRS where extensive model studies will be made for compliance of minimum requirements, and to qualify for animal and/or patient implant, such that the implant operating time be extended to longer durations. The test bench will model the circulatory system of vertebrate / human as prototype, and will provide quantifiable effects on tissues and organs. A test protocol will give statistical information of cumulative effect of stress on tissues and organs to determine the risks of medium and long-term implant. Proper scale ratios between model and prototype (adult human) and scaling capability of the model to be used for smaller prototypes (children, teenager, and vertebrates) will be included.

Also, will be done the analysis of elastic behavior of vessels and quantifying its associated elasticity coefficients, the modeling of three identified forces driving vein's flow, and evaluation of shock waves versus flow wave along the system to comply with due constraints at the boundaries. To have required TAH capacity per individual body weight, ultrasound scans will be performed to multiple healthy males weighing from 30 to 160 Kg in 17 steps as sizes M30 thru M160 and females weighing from 20 Kg to 150 Kg in 17 steps as sizes F20 thru F150.

Parameters to be measured in homologous points of model and prototype are: pressures from large vessels up to and included capillaries, flows, velocities, storage, and elastic forces. The work will include: design, construction, and calibration of the test bench, and left installed in a place accessible to researchers from all over.

ACCOMPLISHMENTS AND SHORTCOMINGS

Background and Significance: We are taking as guidelines the following: "Many of the obstacles remaining to successful implementation of the TAH are similar to those experienced with VADs. While considerable strides have been made in design of the TAH, two main obstacles to clinical success stem from the continued thrombogenic nature of the materials employed in the devices, coupled with the design limitations that continue to require percutaneous lines.

However, the newer devices are being designed without the need for a percutaneous line. The surface thrombogenicity necessitates systemic antithrombotic therapy with the attendant risk of hemorrhage. Major remaining clinical complications with the TAH include infection, hemorrhage, end organ failure, thromboembolism and device dysfunction. Major causes of death with current TAH designs include sepsis, multi-organ failure, neurological death most likely dur to thromboembolism, hemorrhage and problems with device fit.

There is a delicate balance between hemorrhage sequelae and thromboembolism that can be modulated by an-thrombotic therapeutic regimen, which remains to be optimized for most devices." (Expert Panel Review of the NHLBI TAH Program, Vallee L. Willman, Chair. 1998-1999)

PREVIOUS INTENTS

It is of no benefit to list the historical events that take us as to where we are today, with the problem as described above in 1999 because can be found elsewhere, but it is good to summarize the two main lines of research that were followed taking only the source of power used. Those two lines were compressed air and electrical power.

The original Dr. Liotta´s air acting on a diaphragm mostly stop temporarily when in parallel an electrical one was developed, but resurrected with the actual SynCardia, while the electrical remain the most sophisticate with the AbioCor thou too heavy. Both have the problem of patient survival which, with few exceptions, are in the order of little more than a year. Myself, apart from my background in engineering, worked closely with Dr. Kolff and told him to follow the path of electrical power (Annex 3).

Later I designed, applied for a patent, presented it in a Congress (Annex 3) and was adopted and build as AbioCor with the result shown above thank to D. Lederman who, I recall almost for sure, he attended the Congress and asked questions. I waited for some years to expect progress that did not came and concluded that a test bench was required to address those factors that were taken as negligible and address them with a fresh approach to identify in more subtle ways those long-term effects that impede a better performance.
Here are his conclusions and he hope that others, again, can consider to make a contribution in the next practical phases.

PRESENT SITUATION AS OF MIDDLE 2017

Today we reached a point where in more than 20 years has not been surpassed the average one year of TAH implanted survival, with some exceptions probable due to exceptional conditions of the patient.

Therefore, seems appropriate to move un step forward trying to solve the unknowns that make this situation too prevalent.

We think that a test bench to identify problems of small magnitude, which by accumulative effect does not permit go beyond and reach the original goal of a minimum of 5 years survival is inevitable.

A Test Bench is a method that has built the modern world, from supersonic planes, large naval carriers, rocket to the moon and beyond, but seems that physicians have not taken advantage of their expertise but in few cases of medical equipment hardware. The main surprise of those not familiar with their methods find that an analogic model scaled down or up look very different of the real thing and worse, that they use different materials and is incomprehensible how it can provide static or dynamic information?

There a simple reason for that: physics and mathematics are of high grade and only very specialized professional can use it with confidence. In general, are called, as far as to hemodynamics is related Fluid Mechanics Scientists, of course blood is not a fluid but not are neither polluted waters, industrial of many types, non-Newtonian fluid, and so on, that is not obstacle to be called anyway Fluid Mechanics Scientists.

We reach a point in time that a multiple professional team must begin to work jointly without delay, may be the NIH could help by organizing a multidisciplinary effort, because there is no doubt that there is a future for the TAH, as weak it is the argument that there is no future.

Many negative results have been obtained in the last 50 years, but positives too, from few hours of implant to one year or more, tell us something.

THE FUTURE

Please observe that research teams lack contributions of scientists specialized in Fluid Mechanics as used in labs everywhere. I will show now the essential as they could approach the problem of flow in the vascular system.

Therefore, we will address the following subject matters to be taken into consideration:

- Research Designs and Methods
- Criteria for the Transition Volume
- Dimensional Analysis of the General Flow Function
- The elastic behavior of vessels
- Minimum common dimensionless group
- Flow chart for data acquisition and processing
- Data acquisition and processing from model and prototype
- Notes on testing with alternative to blood
- Apparatus to establish laminar flow, equilibrium and conservation of mass.
- How to setup the bench, calibrate, and made tests and studies
- Example of first experiment with Clinical implications

Research Design and Methods

Physics and Mathematics background: Because of the large number of variables in hemodynamic problems, it is almost impossible to develop comprehensive rational relationships to use as the basis to design a TAH instead of a trial and error method. Consequently, the dynamic phenomena need to be studied by using the basic principles of similitude to correlate model and prototype behavior.

The first step to accomplish is to perform a dimensional analysis for homogeneity. Any equation expressing a physical relationship between quantities must be dimensionally homogeneous and numerically equivalent. Dimensional homogeneity states that every term in an equation when reduced to the fundamental dimensions must contain identical powers of each dimension. For a model to predict the true performance of the prototype certain laws of similarity should be observed, i.e., the two flows should be mechanically similar.

Mechanical similarity implies that the physical behavior of the model simulates in a known manner the physical behavior of the prototype, so that the latter can be predicted from the former. Several kinds of similarity are defined as follows:

1. Geometric similarity exists when the ratios of all homologous dimensions on the model and prototype are equal.
2. Kinematic similarity exists when the ratios of all homologous velocities and accelerations are equal in the model and prototype.
3. Dynamic similarity requires that the ratios of all homologous forces (pressure, inertia, gravity, viscosity, elasticity and surface tension) be the same in the model and prototype.
4. Thus, dimensional analysis combined with experimental data aids in the development of design curves and in obtaining a dimensionless relationship between variables. Dimensionless graphs provide equations in non-dimensional form with the advantage that they are independent of the system of units used in performing the experiments. When this point is reached, then the Operation of the Model can be done and Verification of Model-Prototype Conformance.

The basic principles of Fluid Mechanics for blood are: External constraints on the process [conservation of mass, conservation of momentum (linear and angular momentum), conservation of energy, and internal mechanics of the process (increase in energy, space-mass-time dimensional framework). Figure 6 depicts wave route and system boundaries for computational purposes, the transition volume (Fig. 5) is the volume of microcirculation controlled by capillary, surface tension and change in viscosity according the Fahraeus-Lindqvist effect.

For large vessels is assumed to be discontinuous (non-steady flow), because in these vessels continuity will produce the hardening of the vessel walls and tissues over time, and organs will be subject to cumulative strain and malfunction conductive to future collapse. Flow must be unsteady, transient. If it is steady has to change over time to supply the changing body requirements, where the steady state will last for periods of time only.

The transient motion of a pressure wave through a vessel line is occasioned by a change in pressure, the effects associated with this phenomenon depend on the celerity of the pressure wave and may produce severe stresses in the vessel walls or sensitive capillaries at the end of the line. As the wave moves upstream, the flow velocity is reduced. The transmission of a pressure increment wave can be described by the energy and continuity equations.

If it is desired to know the variation of head with time, an any location in the circulatory system, the problem is one of transient flow and an exact analysis is impossible. Therefore, it is necessary to model the system by solving the following equations:

For steady incompressible flow, the equation of continuity is

$$\frac{\delta v_x}{\delta x} + \frac{\delta v_y}{\delta y} + \frac{\delta v_z}{\delta z} = 0$$

The equation of continuity follows from the requirement that the excess mass entering the vessel in a given time increment must equal the increment added to the total mass already within, the latter increment is made possible by stretching the pipe walls. The increase in diameter due to the pressure increment is calculated by integrating the equation of stress in a thin ring.

The work done in stretching the walls is equal to the average force in the wall multiplied by the elongation of the circumference. The latter in turn is the initial circumference times the unit strain. The energy equation is

$$\frac{\delta H}{\delta x} + \frac{fV^2}{D(2g)} = -\frac{1}{g}(\frac{\delta V}{\delta T} + V\frac{\delta V}{\delta x})$$

Neglecting terms, can be written as

$$\frac{\delta H}{\delta x} = -(\frac{1}{g})\frac{\delta V}{\delta T}$$

which is the fundamental equation for surging flows in a flow line.

Criteria for the Transition Volume: The network of conduits in the prototype (human circulatory system) will be made by similitude of flow in graded matrix media in the model. Therefore, the basic problem of blood movement will be to find solutions to Laplace´s Equation (operator nabla squared of head equal to zero).

In cases for which an exact solution might be obtainable, but would be unnecessarily complicated, or when it is not possible to make sufficiently simplifying assumptions about a problem, so that it can be solved by an exact method, it will be solved by an approximate procedure within acceptable dispersion around a true value, or minimum acceptable error.

When considering blood is easily taken into account the influence of the compounded properties of fluid and particles in suspension, by using the following equation:

$$v = -\frac{\kappa g}{\nu}\frac{d\varphi}{ds}$$

where the model matrix's permeability and total mass has the proper ratios to the total mass of capillaries and its mass in the prototype. The basic equation for the flow in the completely confined volume is:

$$\frac{\delta^2\varphi}{\delta x^2} + \frac{\delta^2\varphi}{\delta y^2} = 0$$

and the net outward flux due to the flow in one direction only is:

$$Q = \frac{\delta v_y}{\delta y}\Delta x \Delta y H$$

In the prototype, the total flow per unit time is approximated by

$$Q = \frac{\pi r^4 [P_1 - P_2]}{8\eta L}$$

The amount of blood through the Transition Volume, where φ_1 is the head above the lower boundary, is

$$k_1 \frac{\varphi - \varphi_1}{d_1}\Delta x \Delta y$$

d_1 is Δ_{head}

Detailed math computations are part of the research tasks.

Dimensional Analysis of the General Flow Function: Consider a fluid flowing within or around some kind of boundary surface under the impetus of a differential of potential energy resisted by shear stress at the wall and in the fluid, itself. It is obvious that these resistances will be affected by the roughness of the boundary surface and by the viscosity of the fluid, as well as the nature of the fluid (i.e., its density) and by the geometry of the boundary. Under certain conditions, compressibility of the fluid may affect the flow. One equation can be written in functional form with three basic kind of parameters, these are:

1. Geometric terms describing the flow system boundaries.
2. Kinematic terms defining the flow movement.
3. Dynamic terms representing the types of energy (or force) that may have an internal effect on the process:

a) Kinetic energy (or inertial force). This is always present in a moving fluid, and is specified by the mass density of the fluid.
b) Potential energy. In like manner, the potential energy per unit volume is equal to the force per unit area resulting from the fluid´s pressure and position.
c) Viscous energy (or shear, or friction). Flow is always resisted by internal shearing stresses between fluid particles and at the flow boundaries. The rate of this energy decay depends on the molecular structure of the particular fluid and is specified in terms of the viscosity (or dynamic viscosity). In blood phenomena particles in suspension (hematocrit) are subject to this shear effect, they are critical, and needs a carefully scrutiny on cell damage.
d) Gravitational energy (or weight). All masses respond to a gravitational field.
e) Surface energy (or surface tension). This can be understood as the work required to form a free surface or interface between two fluids against the tendency for mixing and dispersal. This energy plays a role in clogging of ducts and cell colonization of artificial surfaces and be modeled in the test bench.
f) Elastic energy (or compression). Fluids will not resist tension, but they do respond to compressive stresses (i.e., their own fluid pressures) by a reduction in volume and a corresponding storage of elastic energy, in a vessel this energy accomplish work when released. This effect is measured by the bulk modulus of elasticity of the fluid.

<u>The elastic behavior of vessels</u>: The pressure wave leaving the left ventricle by changing over time as transient flow, generates a corresponding change in velocity along the vessels. To account for these changes, the elasticity of large and medium conduits changes in diameter by the elasticity of the walls, such that the velocity when reaching the capillaries change completely its regimen becoming mostly laminar, at lower velocity, but with increased wave length.

This important physical explanation permits the computation of the change of diameter from the beginning of the aorta up to the capillaries as two extreme values, where a simplified law of variation in between can be applied. From that an average change of diameters can be deducted and its associated elasticity coefficients.

Other equations to be used are:

Wave transmission in network, Seddan Principle as applied to pipes

$$V_w = \frac{1}{D}\frac{dQ}{dy}$$

Shock Wave in capillaries

$$(c^2)\delta V$$

because

$$\frac{\delta H}{\delta x} = -(\frac{1}{g})\frac{\delta V}{\delta T} \; or \; \delta H \propto \delta V$$

also

$$\frac{\delta H}{\delta T} = -(\frac{c^2}{g})\frac{\delta V}{\delta x} \; or \; \delta H \rightarrow (c^2)\delta V$$

Condition of minimum TAH power requirement

$$\delta H > 0$$

Suction in an interconnected dual system

$$H = (\frac{p_d}{\gamma} - \frac{p_s}{\gamma}) + (z_d - z_s) + (\frac{v_d^2}{2g} - \frac{v_s^2}{2g})$$

Elasticity quantification related to pressure wave

$$\delta D = \frac{D^2}{2tE_p}\delta p$$

Flow in porous media, Darcy

$$v = -k \frac{\Delta \varphi}{\Delta s}$$

Porous radius R for equivalent capillary:

$$\kappa = \frac{R^2}{8}$$

These last two formulas permit to find the equivalent porous media as function of known radius of capillaries under consideration (see Figure 15).

MINIMUM COMMON DIMENSIONLESS GROUPS

Parameter	Definition	Qualitative ratio effects
Reynolds number	$Re = \dfrac{UL}{\nu}$	$\dfrac{\text{inertia}}{\text{viscosity}}$
Weber number	$We = \dfrac{\rho U^2 L}{\sigma}$	$\dfrac{\text{inertia}}{\text{surface tension}}$
Euler number	$Eu = \dfrac{p - p_o}{\rho U^2}$	$\dfrac{\text{pressure}}{\text{inertia}}$
Drag or lift coefficient	$C_D, C_f = \dfrac{F_D, F_L}{0.5 \rho U^2}$	$\dfrac{\text{drag force, lift force}}{\text{dynamic force}}$
Eckert number	$Ec = \dfrac{U^2}{c_p T_o}$	$\dfrac{\text{kinetic energy}}{\text{enthalpy}}$
Strouhal number	$St = \dfrac{\omega L}{U}$	$\dfrac{\text{oscillation speed}}{\text{mean speed}}$

Where:

Symbol	Quantity	Dimension
L	Length	(L)
U	Velocity	(LT^{-1})
p	Pressure, stress	$(ML^{-1}T^{-2})$
ω	Angular velocity	(T^{-1})
ν	Kinematic viscosity	$(L^2 T^{-1})$
σ	Surface tension	(MT^{-2})
F	Force	(MLT^{-2})
ρ	Density	(ML^{-3})
T	Temperature	(θ)
c_p	Specific heat	$(\theta^{-1} L^2 T^{-1})$

All dimensionless formulas above are commonly used to compare percentage of dispersion out of a known value numbers, generally one [1], such that difficult to measure qualitative effects such as surface tension or enthalpy can be evaluated as function of more accessible parameters. In our case the known values are those of a standard healthy adult male.

Fluid flow involves complex problems which cannot be solved by analytical methods alone and one has to rely on experimental data. To test a device, the performance of the component parts is studied by conducting series of experiments or tests on scale replica (model) of the system (prototype).

The application of dimensional analysis and similitude enables the simplification of experiments and in correlation and interpretation of experimental data. In a Model, alternative designs can be tried before entering a costly undertaking. Alternative designs are referred to the Test Research Station (TRS) where extensive model studies are made for compliance of minimum requirements.

The research plan is to build a TRS with the tasks of developing Geometric, Kinematic and Dynamic Similarities of the Systemic and Pulmonary systems, adjust wave propagation and pressure distribution in the system, and develop Protocols for Flow, Pressure, Velocities, Capillary Rise and Elastic Forces.

A basic theory of the phenomenon and the existence of adequate data are required for successful model testing. Model testing has stimulated research, design, and performance prediction work. Therefore, a TRS will be built to test developed TAHs to qualify for animal and / or patient implant, such that the patient survival be extended to a desirable 5 years' minimum.

Application of pulsed continuous-flow technology can help in solving some of these issues and is currently being applied in the research towards a new generation of devices.

THE TEST BENCH METHOD

The TRS will model the circulatory system of vertebrate / human as prototype, and will provide quantifiable effects on tissues and organs. A test protocol will give statistical information of cumulative effect of stress on tissues and organs to determine the risks of medium and long-term implant.

The TRS will operate with synthetic blood per its physical characteristics, and will be driven by a two-way variable flow pump in a closed circuit for continuity and several needed studies like suction and walls elasticity of veins and arteries.

Out of the complexity of the project it is possible to see how simple the overall scheme looks like in the following graph:

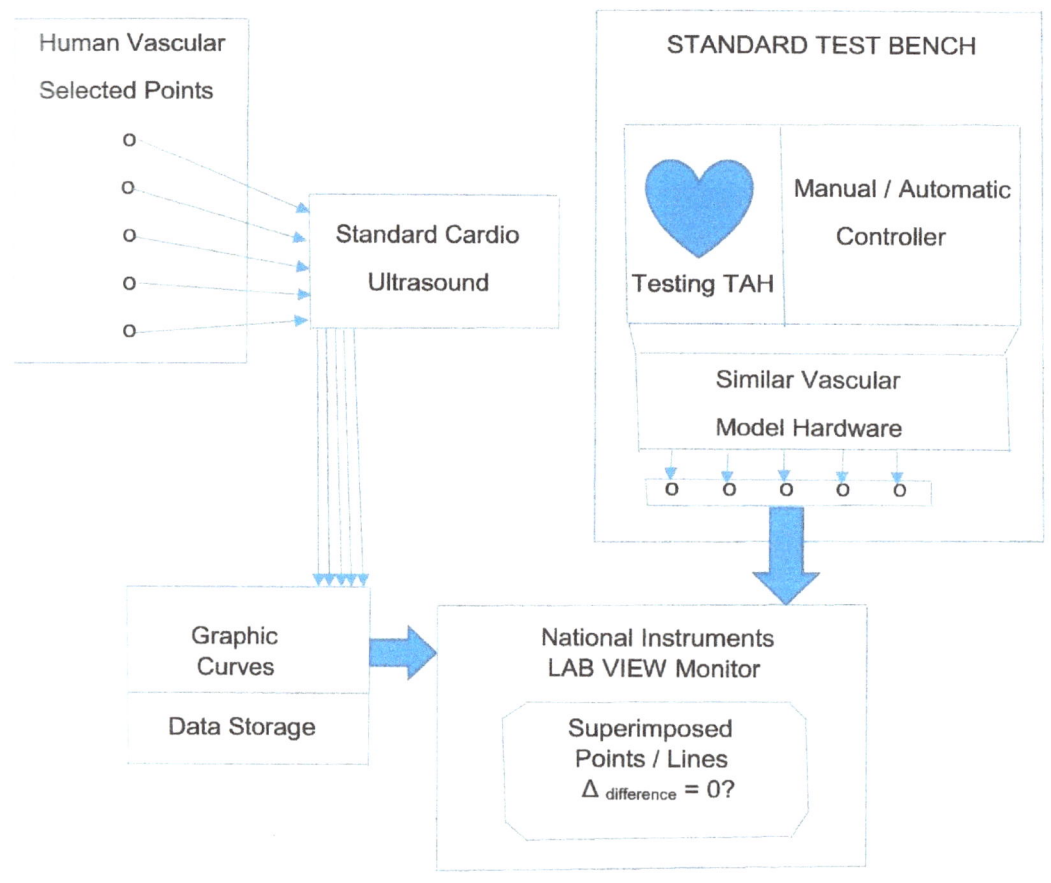

To have required TAH capacity per individual body weight and height, ultrasound scans will be performed to multiple healthy males weighing from 30 to 160 Kg in 17 steps as sizes M30 thru M160 and females weighing from 20 Kg to 150 Kg in 17 steps as sizes F20 thru F150.

Additionally, evaluation and experiments with the actual TRS will be initiated to see if the installation can provide assistance for Clinical use.

TEST RESEARCH STATION COMPONENTS

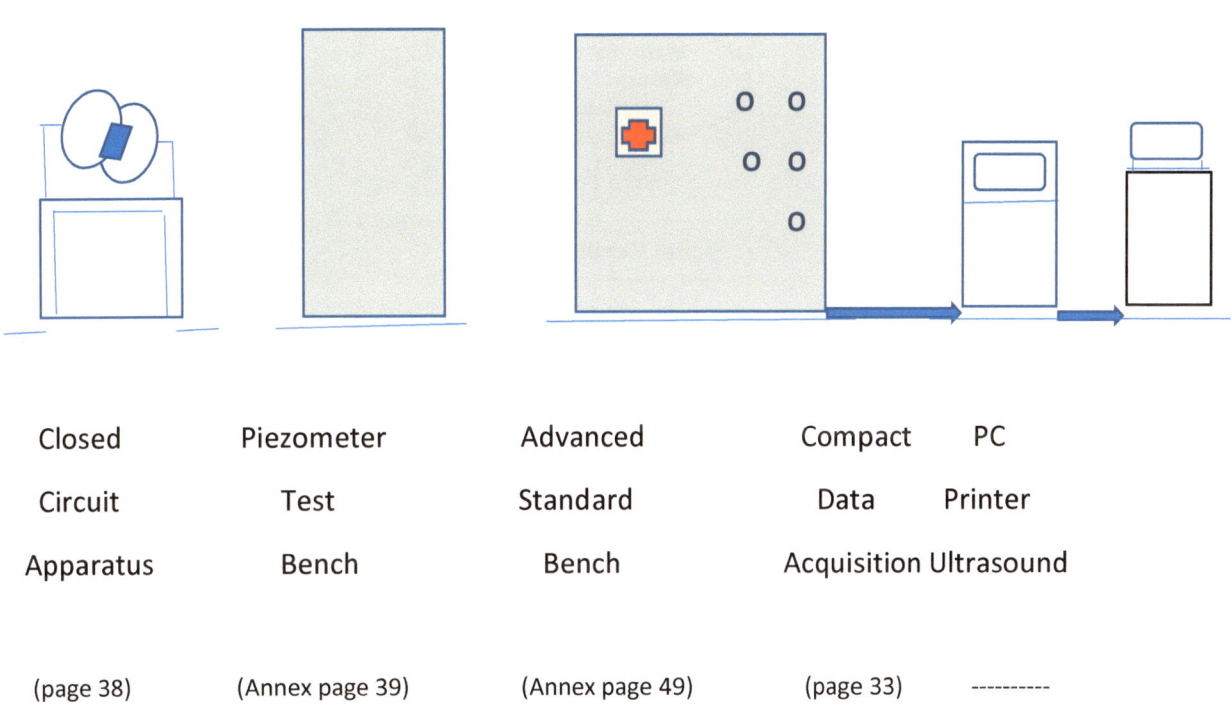

Closed Circuit Apparatus	Piezometer Test Bench	Advanced Standard Bench	Compact Data Acquisition	PC Printer Ultrasound
(page 38)	(Annex page 39)	(Annex page 49)	(page 33)	----------

The bench will be a unique piece of equipment operated for specific size and weight of patient by exchanging parts to cover the range of the data acquired in an early operation of ultrasound scanning of healthy individuals. Dual pumps will operate de bench to calibrate it to have a threshold of data to serve as basis for comparison with proposed TAH, and discrepancies or compliance.

FLOW CHART FOR DATA ACQUISITION AND PROCESSING

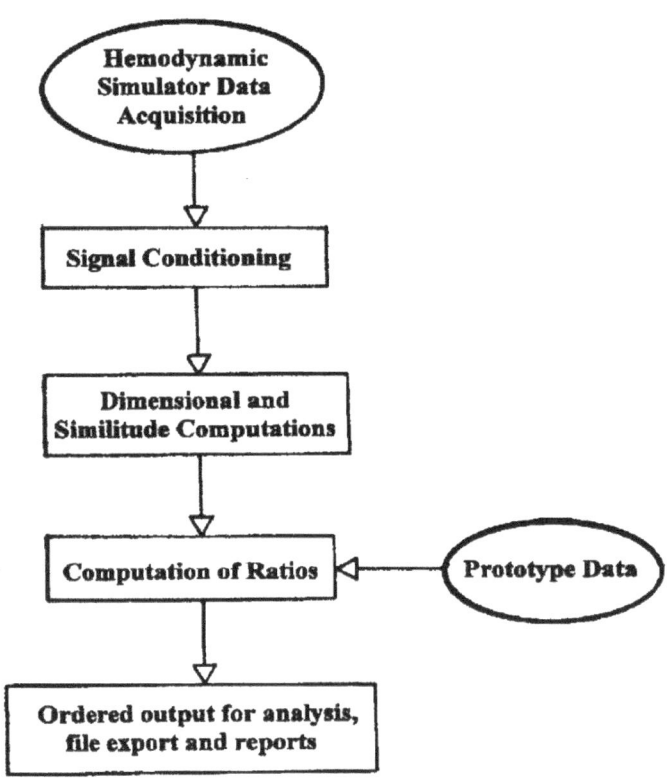

DATA ACQUISITION AND PROCESSING FROM MODEL AND PROTOTYPE

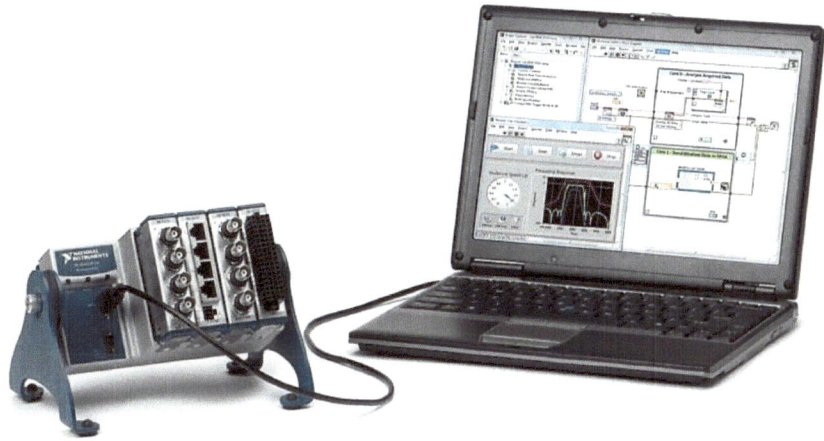

CompactDAQ Acquisition of data from sensors and signals integrates with software LabVIEW for analysis, recording and visualization, both from National Instruments (NI)

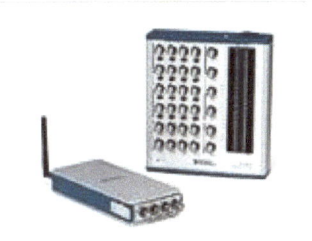

Data acquisition hardware multifunctional with bus USB for low quantity of channels.

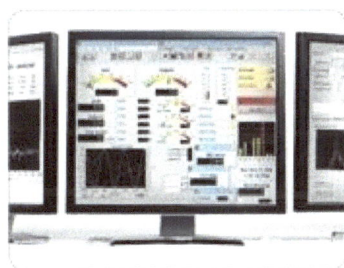

Programable software LabView to monitor comparable data-in from model and prototype.

Notes on testing with alternative fluid flow of natural human blood

Regarding the fluid flow to use in the Bench, there are three options: water, blood or an artificial substitute. Each have its pros and cons.

Water:

Pro = easy to use

Con = it is Newtonian differing of non-Newtonian blood. Requires additional work without advantages.

Blood:

Pro = If possible, the best option.

Con = Difficult to handle, requiring extra labor to clean the Bench. Few runs will be made for comparison with techniques and alternatives made up to a time when will be advisable to check precision.

Substitute of Blood / Synthetic / Alternative:

Pro = A Blend can be made where viscosity can be calculated (e.g., Refutas three steps Equation), and/or lab simplified viscometer by contrast of actual blood vs blend. Nonetheless, three passes in the calibration process (Apparatus, Piezometer and Standard Bench) will give a measurable acceptable analogy with minimum operational error.

Con = Extra work to experiment the better fluids, transport particulates, and correlate properly to actual blood.

MATERIAL FOR ARTERIES AND VEINS: It is not critical but the first material to test must be Silicone.

Test Bench Operations General Planning

Could made in three stages: Build and operate as described above with any pump, upgrade to operate with proposed TAH for compliance, and get approval for animal and human implants.

Deliverables

Upon completion of the Project a Clinic will maintain a "TEST RESEARCH STATION" including the Deliverables of the Project as follows:

(i) Standard Test Bench with documentation of parts installed and drawings as built.

(ii) Software documentation, back up electronic storage files.

(iii) Operations and Maintenance Manual, including failure / error management.

(iv) Written records of the 12 months' setup and finished project.

(v) Calibration standards and other specifications for operating the installation.

Example of two **EXPERIMENTS WITH CLINICAL IMPLICATIONS**

(Directly with the first setup of the Test Bench)

Though the main goal with a TAH Test Bench is evaluate efficiency of a proposed TAH, has been suggested to use it for vascular studies. In general once in operation the Test Bench, it will be available to the professional community to propose or carried out the study, simulation or analysis of specific cases.

Because it is set to TAH and no other situations, if a problem can be solved as it is the set will be fine, otherwise if it requires modification of the Bench, then that modification must be carried out properly. Here we show two very simple case to verify if *it is correct as proposed:*

(1) ATRIAL FIBRILLATION STUDY APPLYING HIGH PRESSURE ON THE SYSTEM

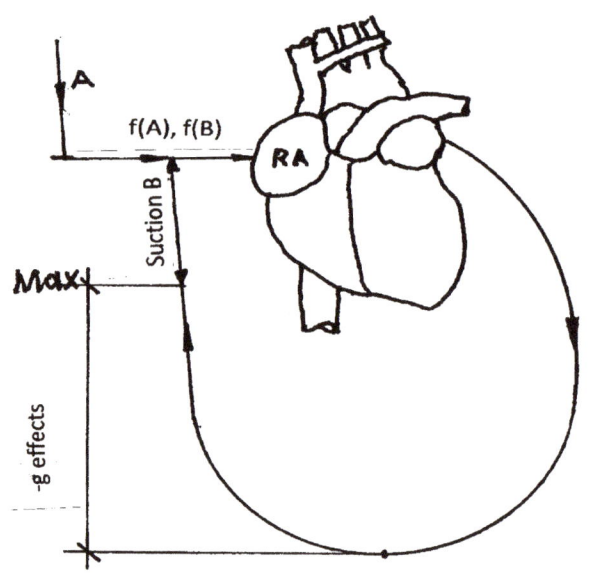

By pressuring on any part of the system while running in stable equilibrium in the test bench, and no taken into account brain control, the system will become unstable showing an analogy to fibrillation as it varies on time once initiated.

By measuring the variation of current (amperes) by the pumps' motors in a lapse of time will be possible to obtain a quantification.

In the extreme if **f(A) + f(B) < 0** the right atrium will work partially or not at all and, in the bench: the motor will accelerate out of control resembling a collapsing heart. There is indetermination if **f(A) + f(B) = 0**

If brain control is overwhelmed by rapid and changing arriving information, its response could be not enough efficient despite the high velocity of the nervous signal, and the heart will behave erratic and in the extreme to stop working. By applying an electric shock to a patient, the whole phenomena reset and start all over with a degree of success proportional to the seriousness of the problem.

If the stable equilibrium of circulation in the two-interconnected circuit is broken, it appears prima-facie, that alteration is what trigger fibrillation, be it a disturbance originated by physical, chemical or biological action.

If **f(A) + f(B) > 0 or f(A) – f(B) > 0** there will be not fibrillation as far as pressure is related.

MAX in the diagram above means equilibrium by the principle of the communicating vessels minus head losses occurring between pipe inlet point up to that Max level which is never the same as the level at the inlet point.

2) THE VENTRICLE's MUSCLE SUCTION FACTOR

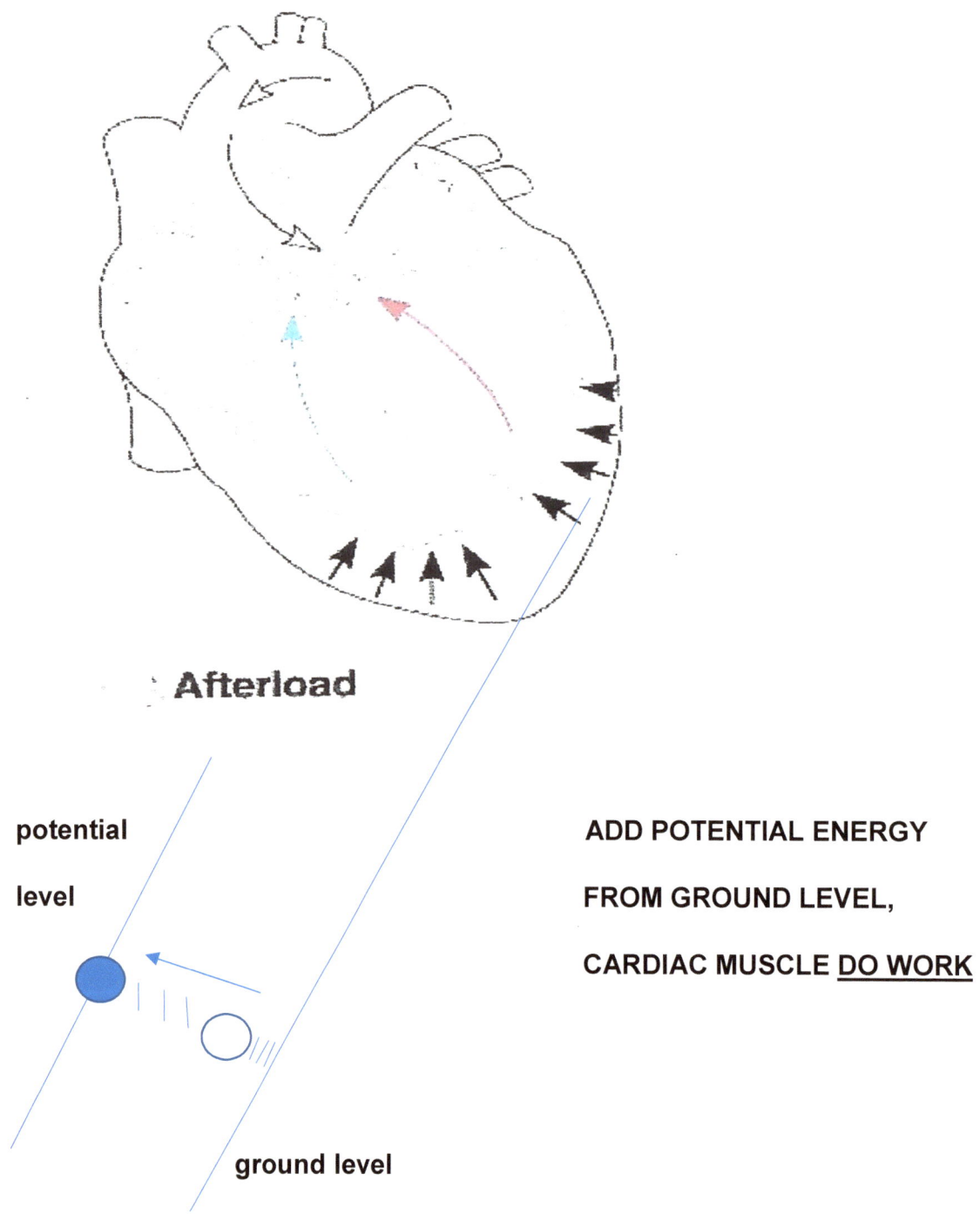

Afterload

potential level

ground level

ADD POTENTIAL ENERGY FROM GROUND LEVEL, CARDIAC MUSCLE <u>DO WORK</u>

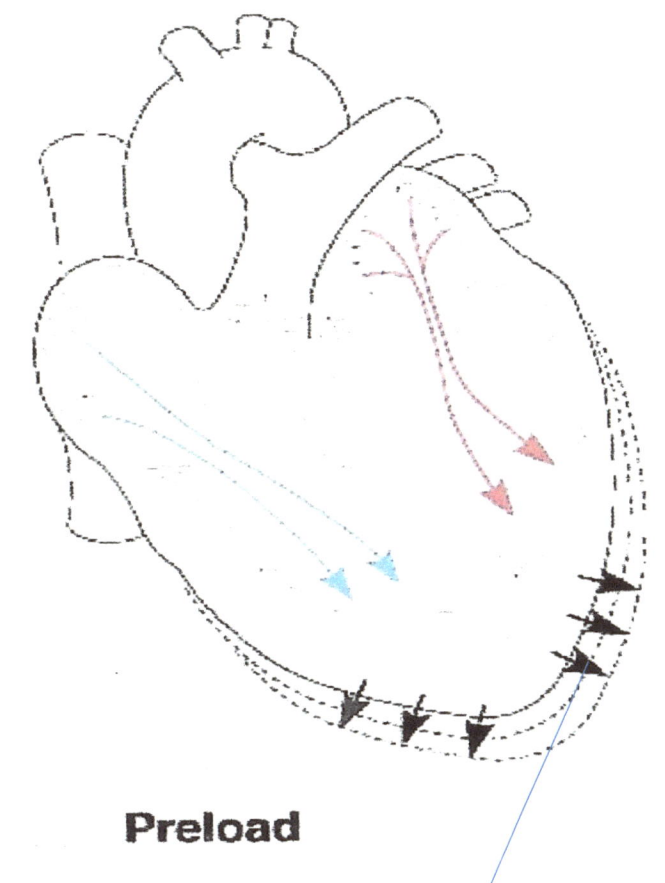

Preload

Potential level

ground level

RETURN TO GROUND LEVEL RELEASE KINETIC ENERGY, <u>DO</u> SUCTION <u>WORK</u>, ITS CONTRIBUTION TO FILL ATRIA AND VENTRICULES ARE RELEVANT

GUIDELINES FOR A 3th GENERATION OF TAH

Moving Blood Flow in an Electromagnetic Field

Now with electric power available it is time to advance ahead and try the electromagnetic field to avoid motor, more parts, or compressed air.

First job is to build a unit with the following specifications to test its working, be it solenoid type or linear array as proven technology (motor stator-rotor concept) or other, if any, best suited.

Operates by running its length alternatively back and forth at increasing from zero, constant and decreasing velocities up to zero, repeating the cycle continuously constant, except if electromagnetic field change to a new regime, and once again as stipulated in a protocol for a specific and well define patient per classification as shown in Annexes.

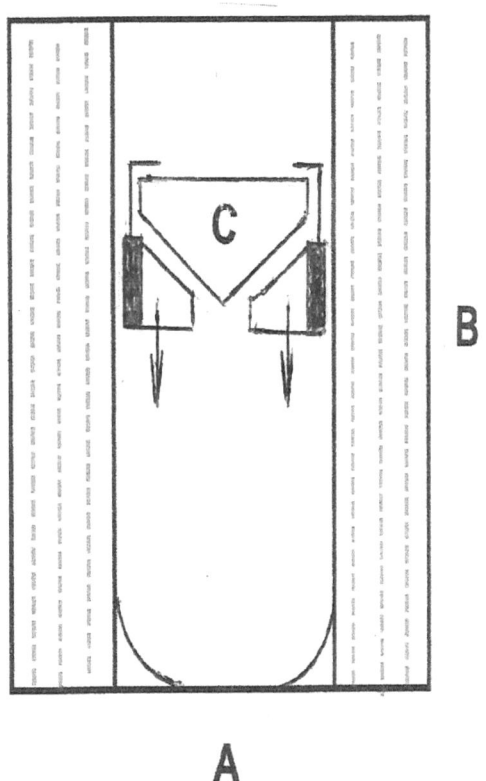

Coil wires: as appropriated

Bio Materials, Carbon Fiber or Plastic: main body and ducts

A = reduced diameter for optimum suction

B = 2.5 in

C = free fly ring (ferromagnetic)

Travel time per run = 1 sec

Volt = 12 V

Power = 5 watts

Max Weigh Total as shown = 180 grams

SMOOTH FLOWING OF BLOOD, PULSATIL SYNCHRONIZATION

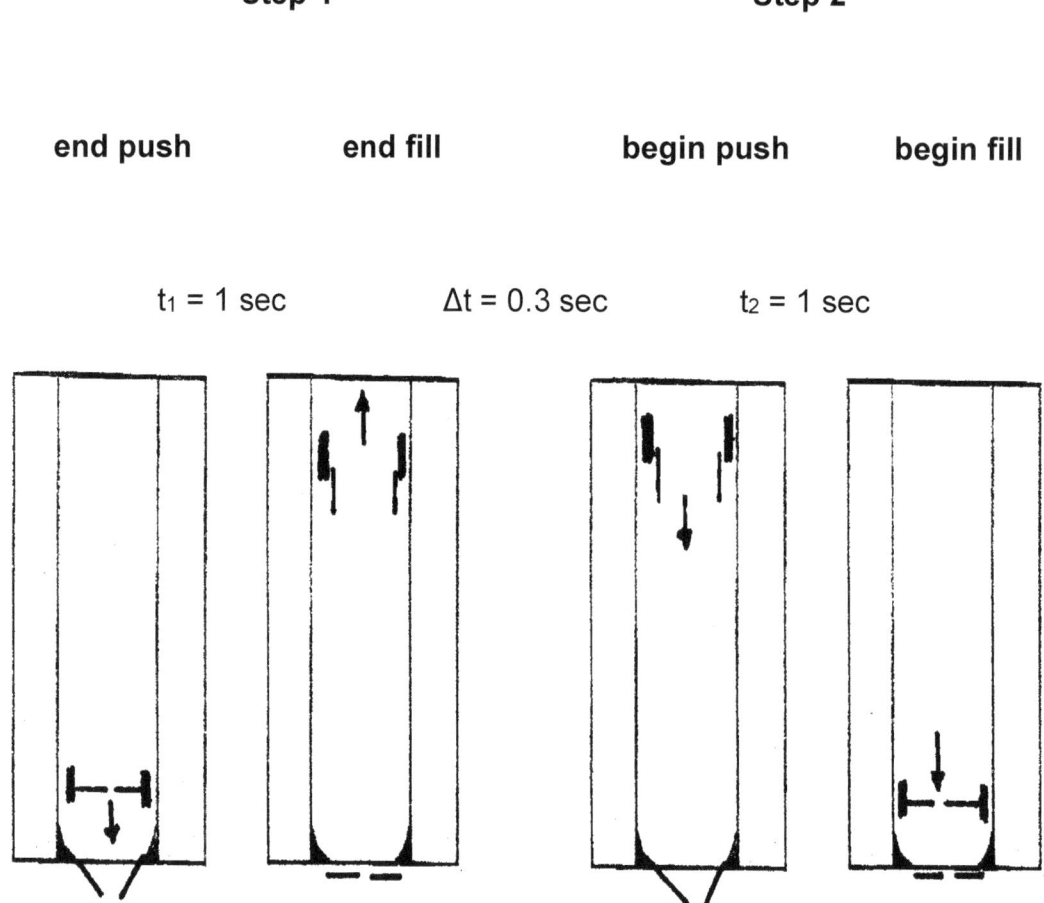

Note that running the full length we have in the circuitry pulse and wave, other type of operation may produce smooth flow but not convenient relative pressure distribution between the systemic and pulmonary circulation.

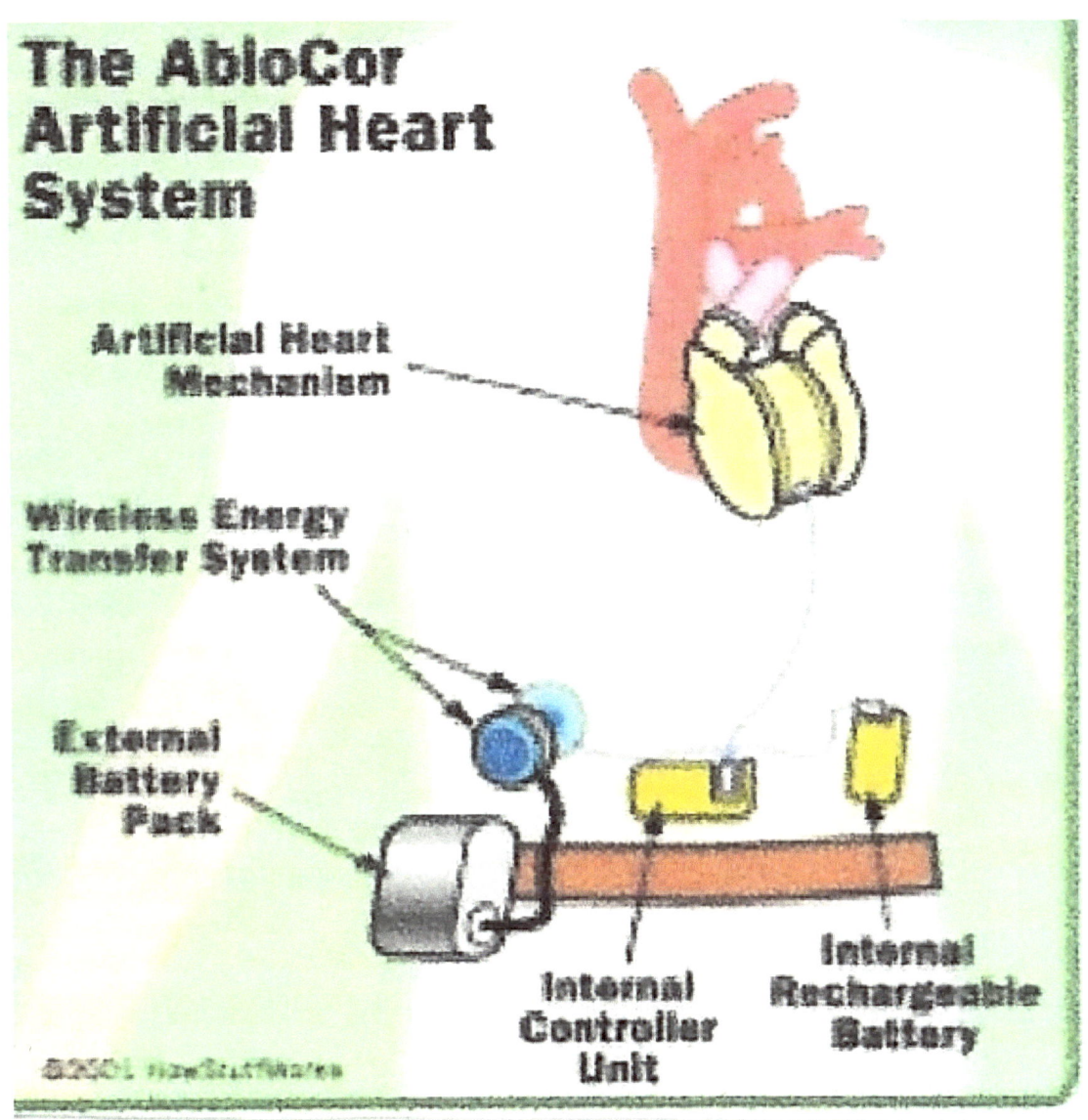

Transcutaneous energy transfer to take as final if no better found.

ANNEX 1

	Page
Figure 1: Main Network Prototype	35
Figure 2: Systemic and Pulmonary Circulation	36
Figure 3: Two Interconnected Closed Circuits	37
Figure 4: The Piezometer Bench	38
Figure 5: Acting Forces in the Piezometer Bench	39
Figure 6: Pressure Wave Route Diagram	40
Figure 7: Synchronized Pumps Principle	41
Figure 8: Power, Flow and Circulation	41
Figure 9: Assemble a TAH	42
Figure 10: Location of Pumps in Vivo	43
Figure 11+12: TAH Pump Replica + Oxygen and Effort	44
Figure 13: TAH Control System by Breathing Rhythm	45
Figure 14: Vessel Branching and Capillaries Analogy	46
Figure 15: Strainer in Line	47
Figure 16: Standard Hemodynamic Simulator	48
Figure 17: Out to Perform by Replica	49
TRS Setup and Operation	50
Exhibit 1: Equations of Similitude for the Test Bench (p.1)	51
Exhibit 2: Protocol for Calibration of the Test Bench (p.2)	52
Exhibit 3: Protocol for Calibration of the Test Bench (p.3)	53
Exhibit 4: Analysis of Risks and Scheme for Analysis	54
Exhibit 5: Form Ultrasound screening for males	56
Exhibit 6: Form Ultrasound screening for males	57

ABOUT HOMOLOGOUS POINTS

MAIN NETWORK PROTOTYPE WITH FLOW DIRECTIONS

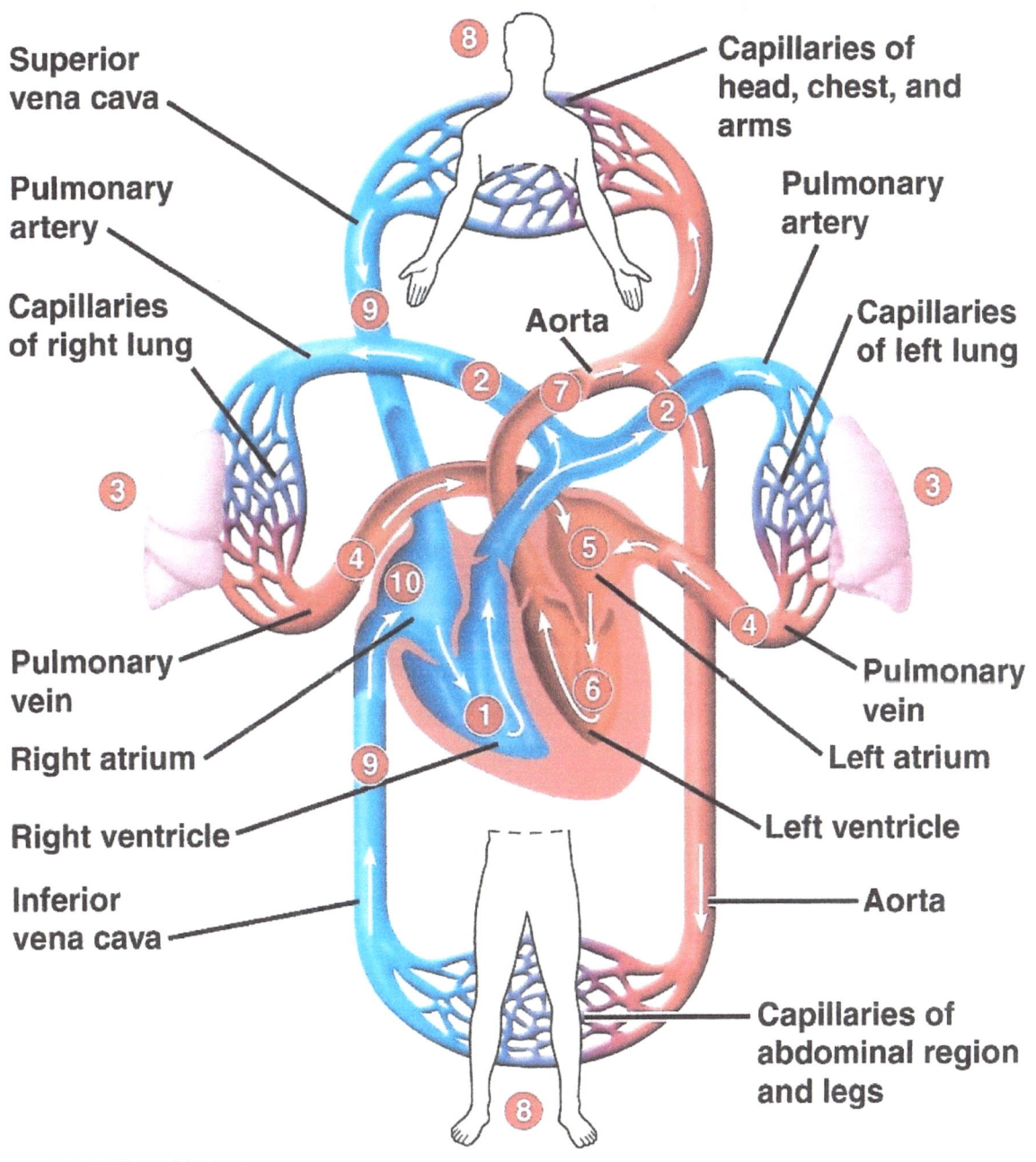

Figure 1

SYSTEMIC AND PULMONARY CIRCULATION

(candidates as homologous points from prototype)

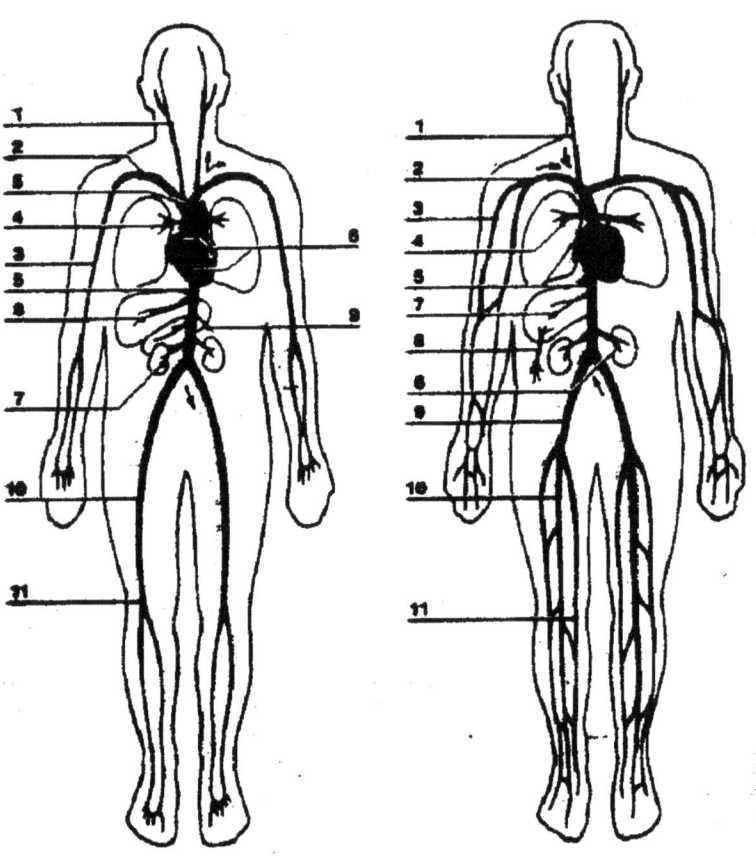

MAJOR ARTERIES	MAJOR VEINS
1 Carotid	1 Jugular
2 Subclavian	2 Subclavian
3 Brachial	3 Cephalic
4 Pulmonary	4 Pulmonary
5 Aorta	5 Vena Cava
6 Coronary	6 Renal
7 Renal	7 Hepatic
8 Hepatic	8 Hepatic Portal
9 Gastric	9 Iliac
10 Iliac	10 Femoral
11 Femoral	11 Great Saphenous

Figure 2

BASIC CONCEPT OF TWO INTERCONNETED CLOSED CIRCUITS

Let us build an apparatus to understand and practice equilibrium under mass conservation

APPARATUS FOR EQUILIBRIUM, CONSERVATION OF MASS AND SYNTHETIC BLOOD

Two Pumps I, II and two Flows $Q_1 = Q_2$

Controller System = Flowmeters Q_i and Valves V_i

Two Interconnected Circuits $(1 - 3)$ and $(2 - 4)$.

$V_1 = k * V_2$ and $k = \Omega_2 / \Omega_1$ where Ω = cross section of pipe

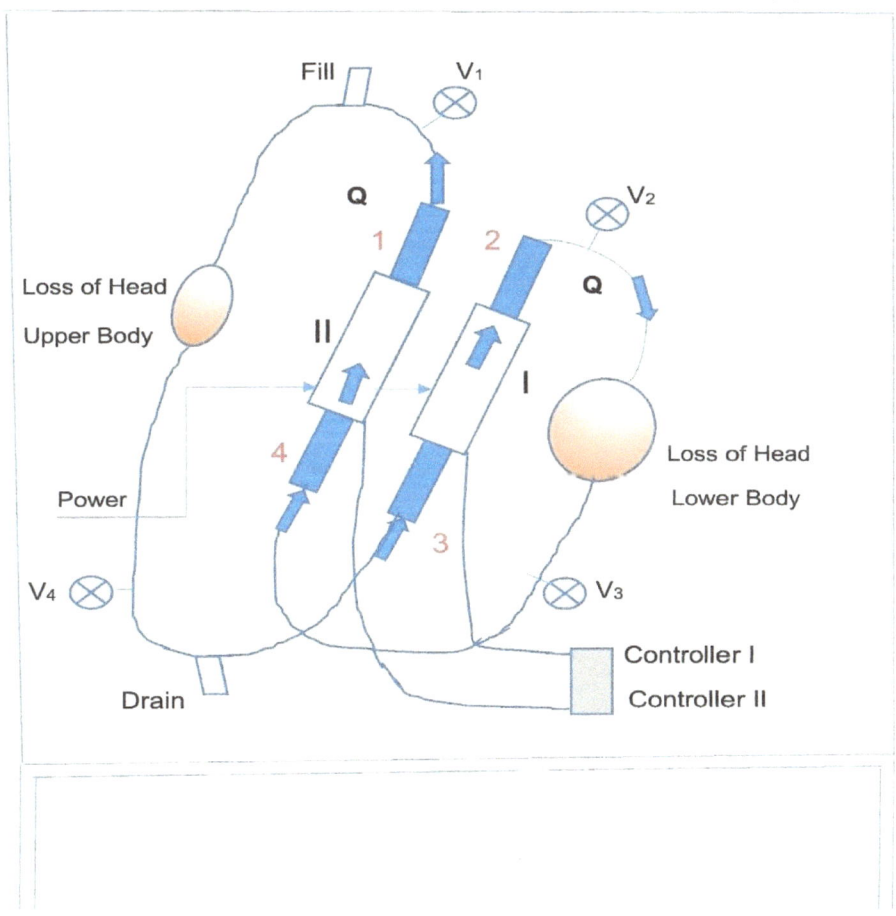

Anybody working in cardiovascular circuitry is or must be, an efficient operator of this type of closed circuit.

Figure 3

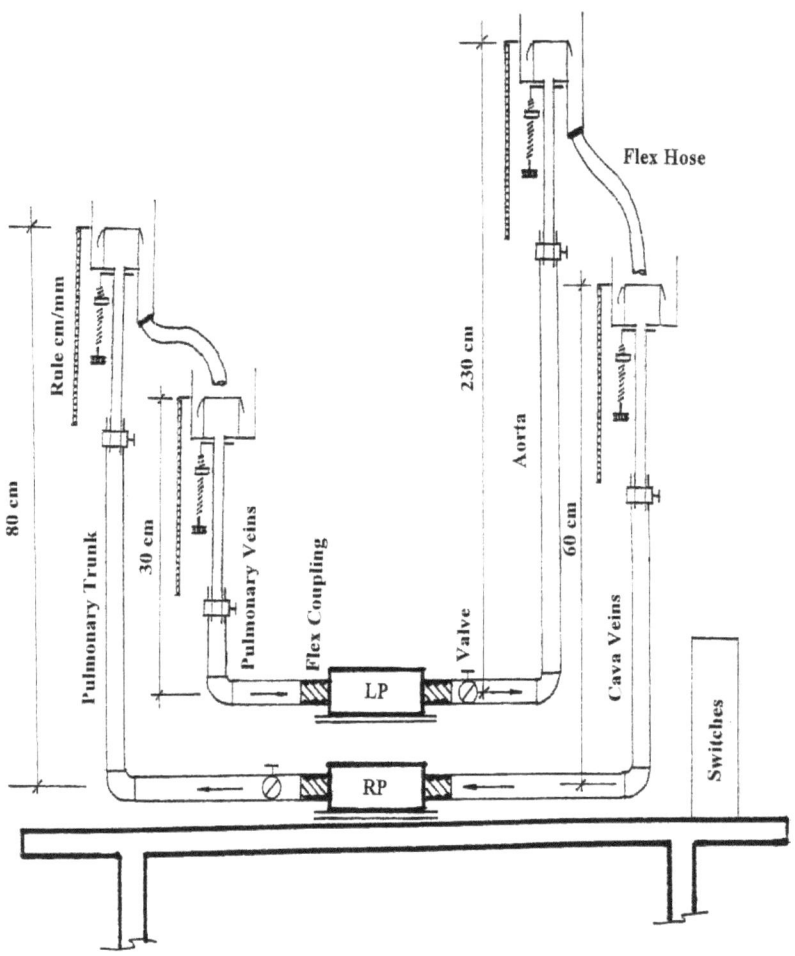

Anybody working in cardiovascular circuitry is or must be, an efficient operator of this type of open circuit where there is variable mass over time to quantify mass gain and losses to analyze unsteady flow and its consequences.

Figure 4

ACTING FORCES IN THE PIEZOMETER BENCH

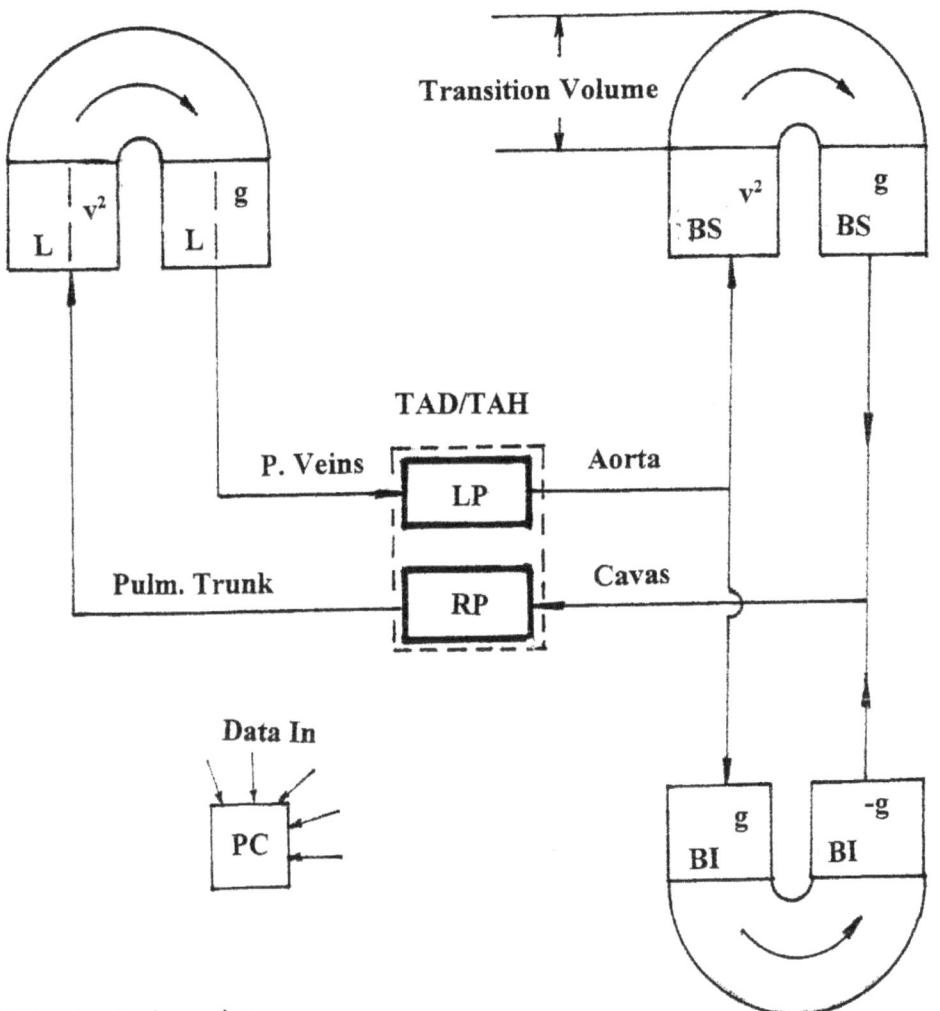

BS: Body Superior
BI: Body Inferior
v^2, g, -g: Predominant Forces

Figure 5

Pressure Wave Route Diagram

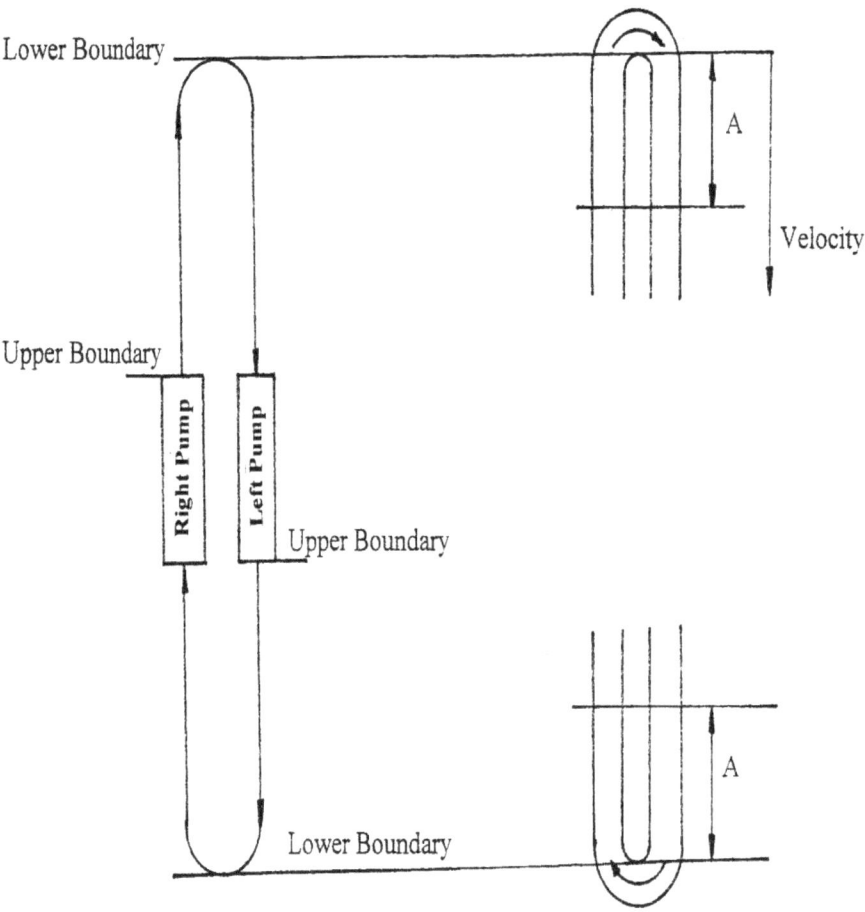

Figure 6

BASIC CONCEPT

Two Synchronized Pumps Principle

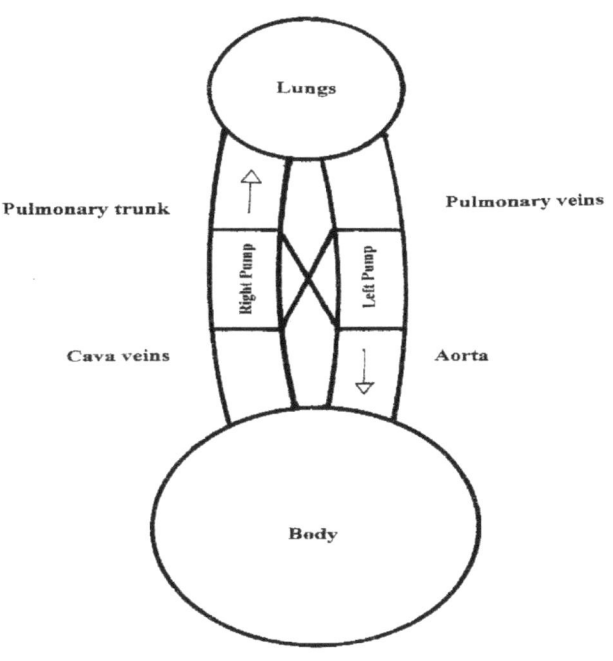

Figure 7

POWER, CONTROL AND FLOWS CIRCULATION IN THE PIEZOMETER BENCH

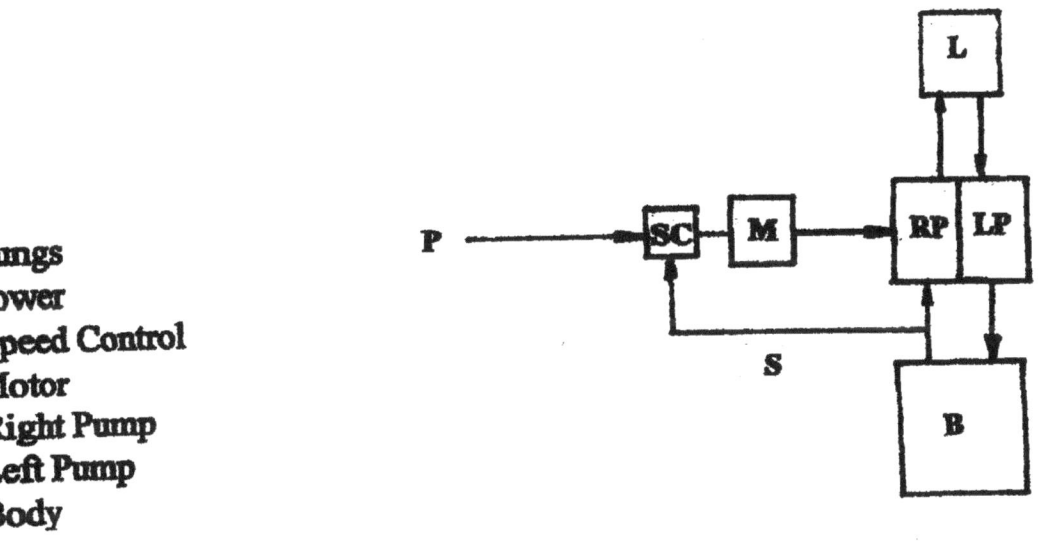

L: Lungs
P: Power
SC: Speed Control
M: Motor
RP: Right Pump
LP: Left Pump
B: Body
S: Signal

Figure 8

Assembled as a hypothetical TAH to evaluate (main suggestion).

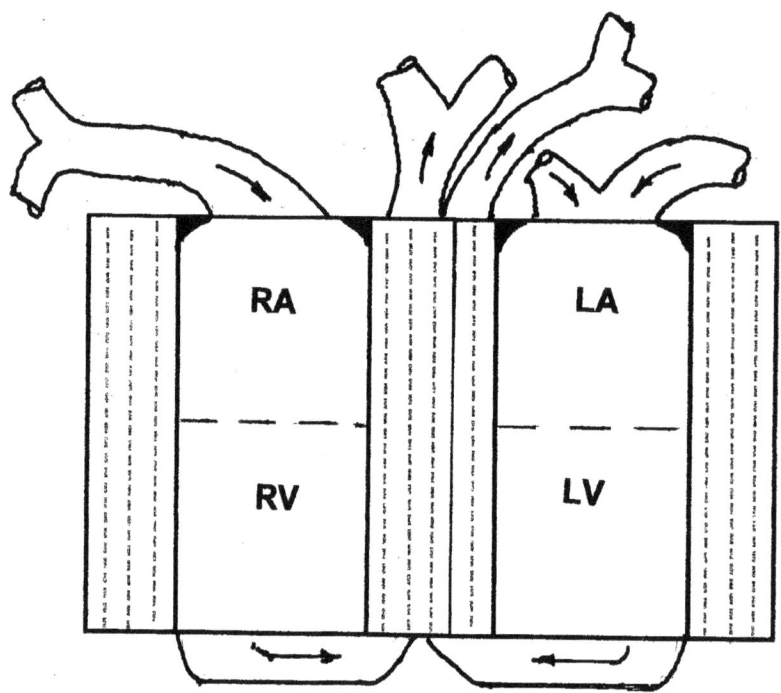

In this scheme, the ascending pipes are located between the two main bodies spaces because they are in contact by a single line. Defined blood volume move by the cylinder (piston or ring) synchronized with its opposing companion such that a continuous pulsatile regime is obtained along the vascular system from a minimum for survival or at rest, up to a maximum, where variation is controlled by the breathing rhythm of a trained patient to perform adequately, and the variation is a consequence of the electric current properly modulated only, following the criteria of simplicity and lightness.

Figure 9

LOCATION OF PUMPS IN VIVO

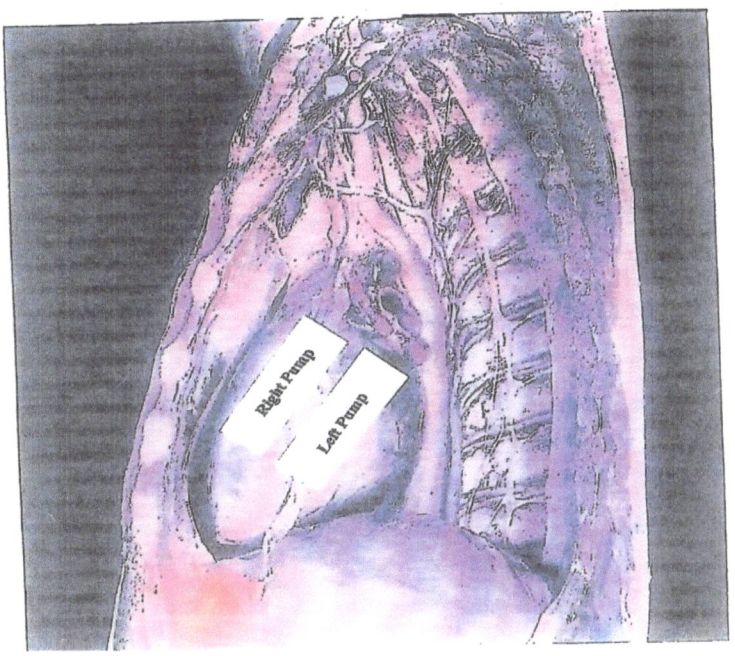

Figure 10

TAH Pump Replica

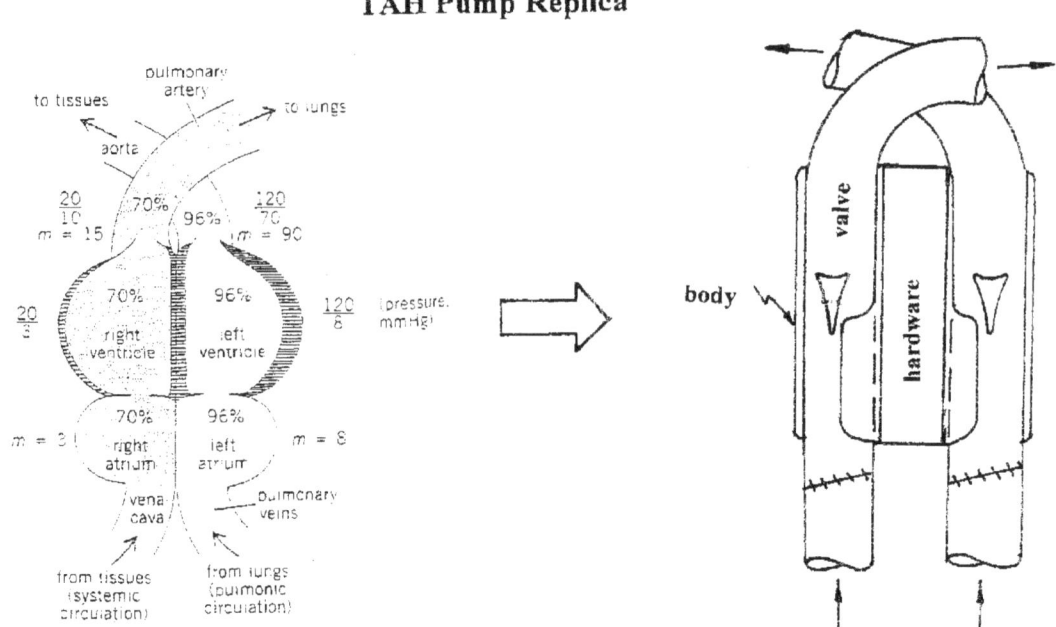

Figure 11

Relation Between Oxygen Required, Effort, and Pump Output

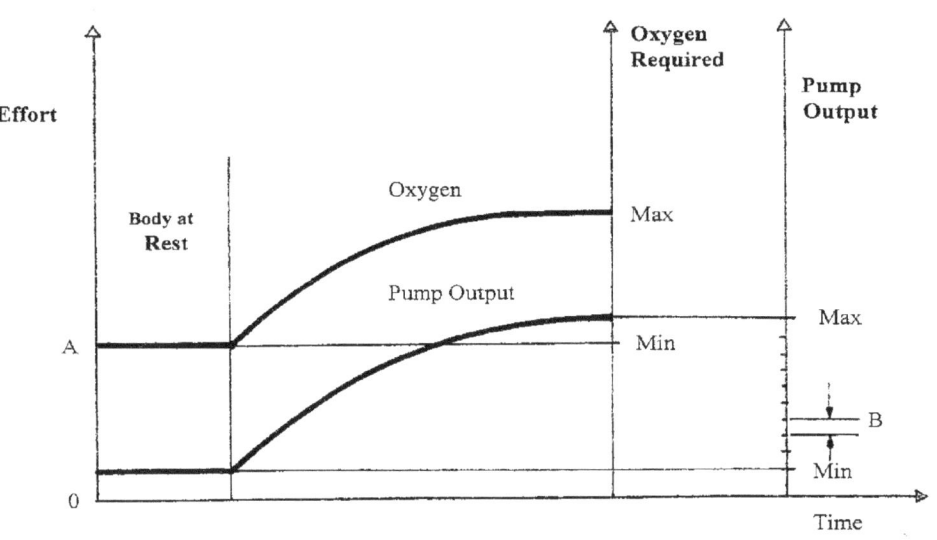

A: start of body effort

B: pump reaction time / output step

Figure 12

AUTOMATIC CONTROL OF TAH BY BREATHING RATE

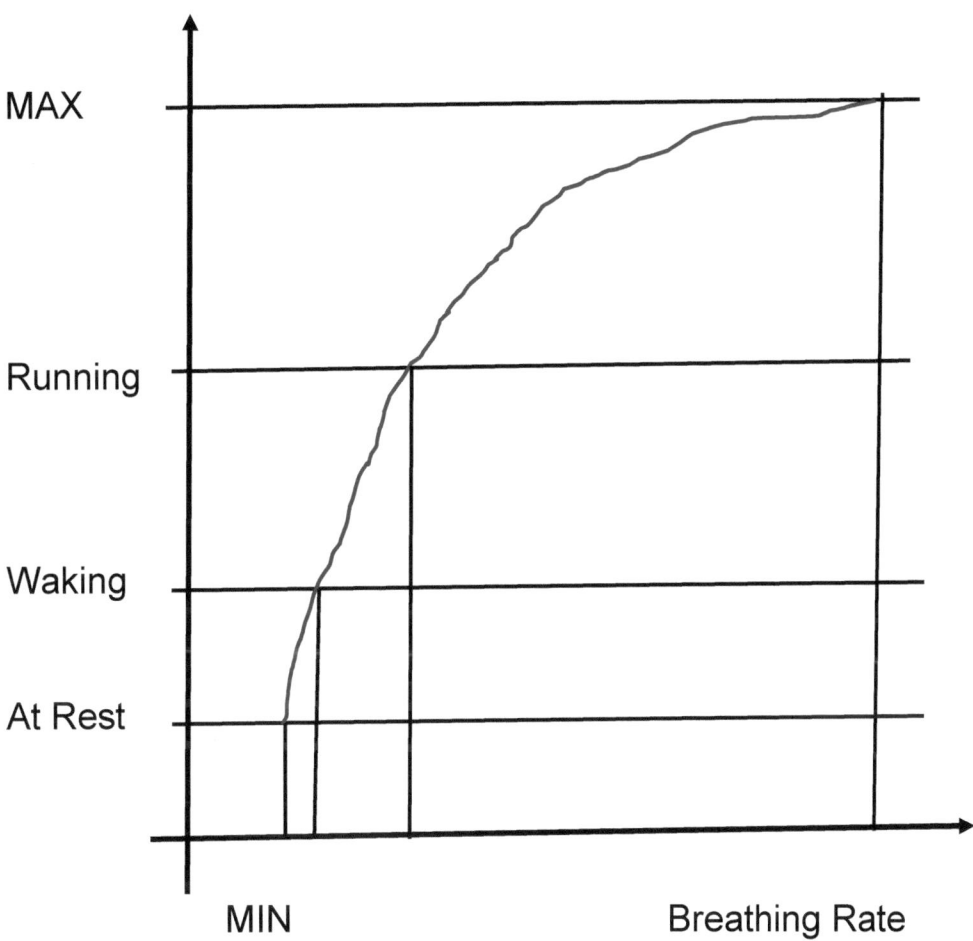

Figure 13

Vessel Branching and Capillaries Analogy

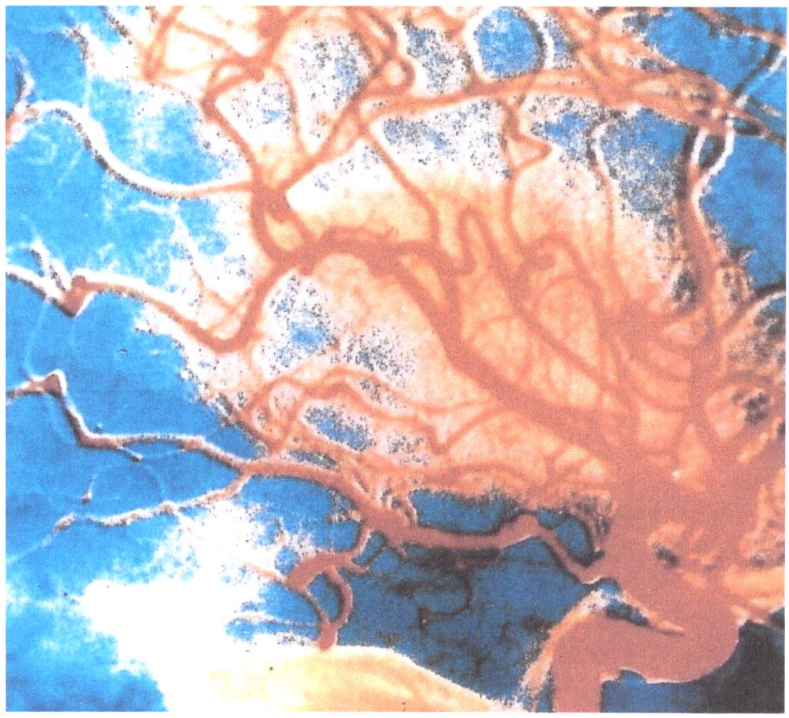

Blood volume in tissues

It is suggested to use a strainer with porous material proportional to part of blood volumes in tissues, installing as many strainers as needed located in proper points of the model to match those homologous points in the prototype as far as to physical properties we refer to, even if the geometry of model and prototype are not congruent.

Figure 14

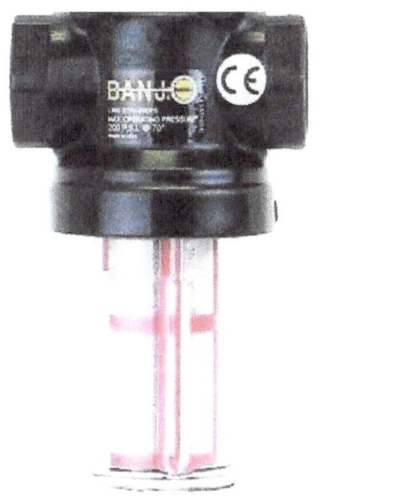 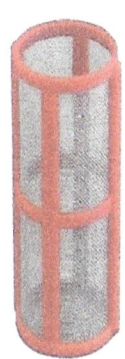

Strainer in line and basket to fill with porous material for velocity flow reduction, where potential is $v^2 / 2g$.

Figure 15

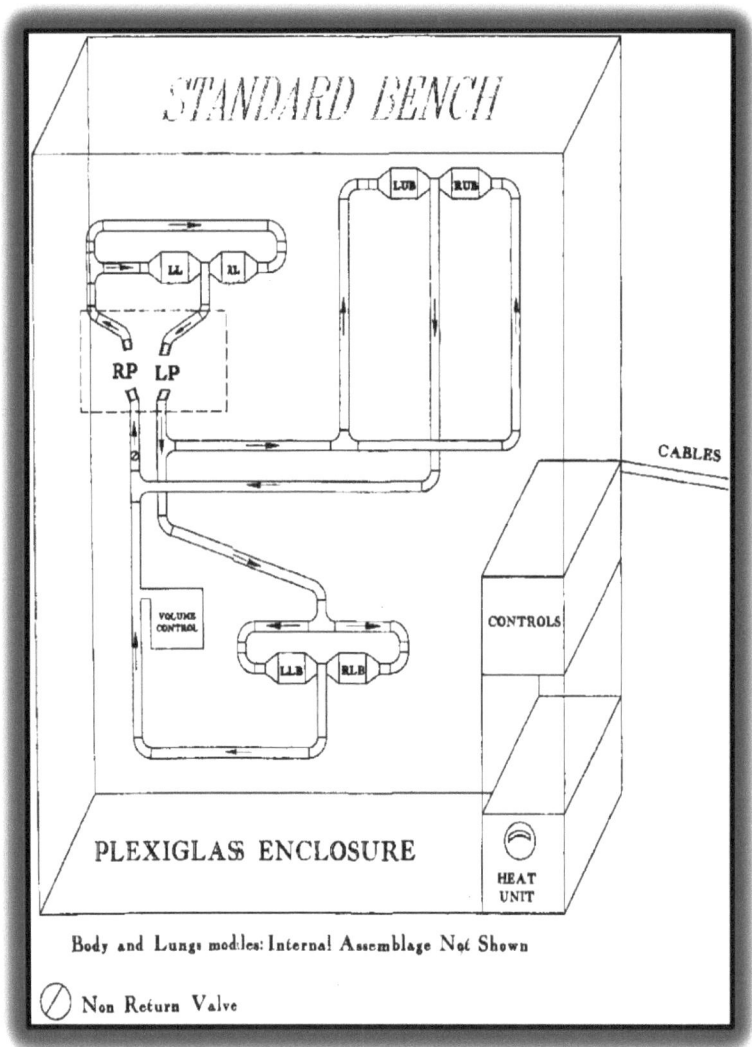

STANDARD HEMODYNAMIC SIMULATOR

This is an old option to be revised, included here to show parts and components.

Figure 16

Output To Perform by Replica

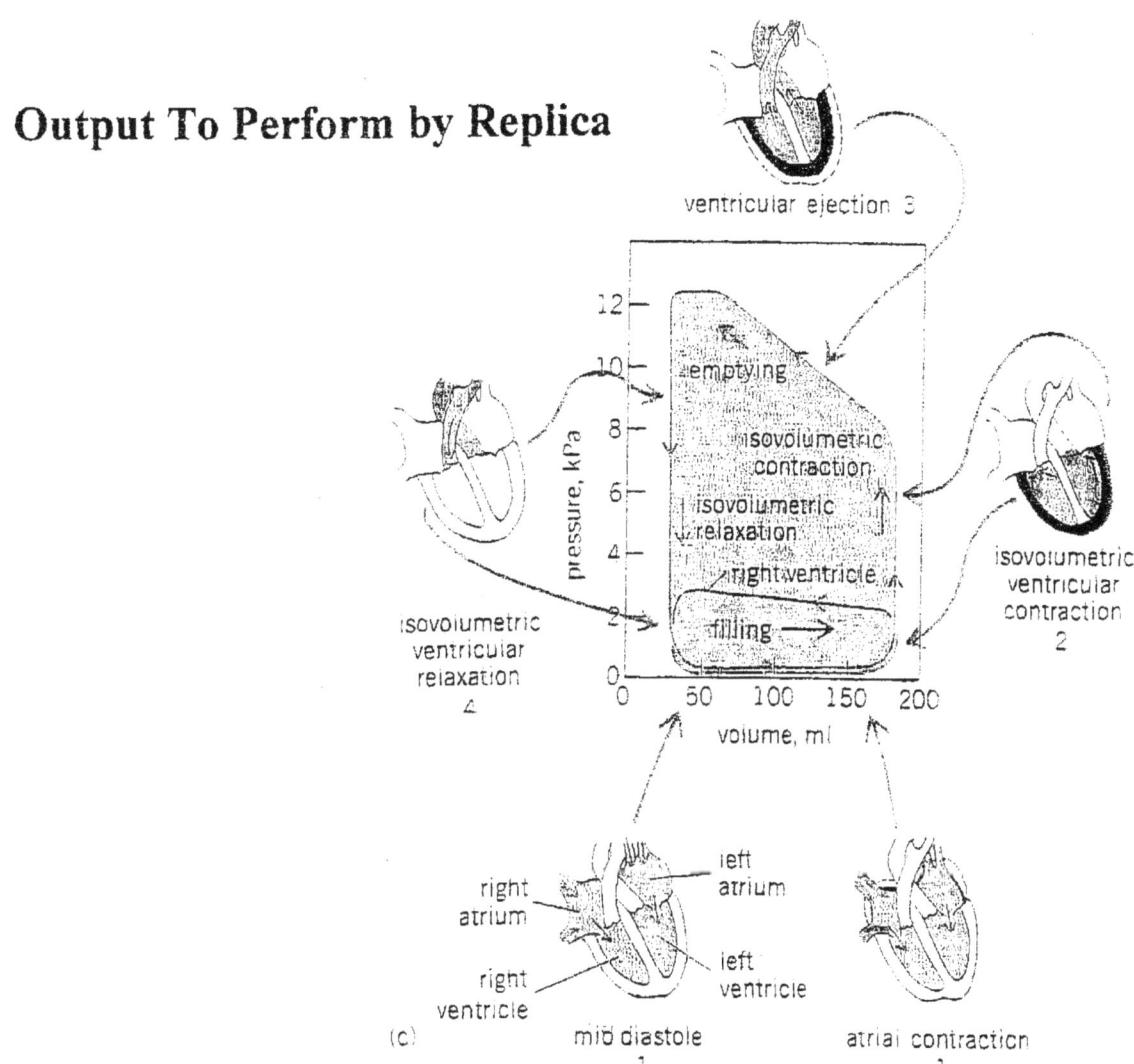

Figure 17

How to set up the Bench for a TAH verification

Run with the dual pump, adjust all controls to operate for a desired body weight and height of an individual.

Once in equilibrium, laminar flow will prevail except inside the TAH and conservation of mass will exist. Check data out is working and curves are displayed in the monitor.

Stop the run, secure the system remain full of fluid.

Disconnect the dual pump.

How to set up the Bench for a clinical study

Run with the dual pump, adjust all controls to operate for a desired body weight and height of an individual.

Once in equilibrium, laminar flow will prevail except inside the pumps and conservation of mass will exist. Check data out is working and curves are displayed in the monitor.

Stop the run, secure the system remain full of fluid.

Disconnect the dual pump.

How to test a submitted TAH

Adjust all controls to operate for a desired body weight and height of an individual. Test in the Apparatus the TAH submitted, reading instruments for continuity, then do the same in the open to the atmosphere Piezometer Bench, watching there are no changing levels in the upper two open recipients to complain with stable equilibrium, continuity, and conservation of mass.

How made a clinical study

Proceed to perform the operation in the Standard Bench by setting the parameters provided by the researcher and follow his/her instructions for how many simulations are instructed to do.

When the operations ends keep the data out in electronic storage, and release the same to the clinical researcher.

End runs. Secure the system remain full of fluid.

Exhibit 1

BASIC TEST BENCH EQUATIONS OF SIMILITUDE

		Equation of model to Match the prototype	Adjusted output under calibration	
Geometry		$L_R = x_p/x_m = y_p/y_m = z_p/z_m$	$L_R = 1$	Matching factors
		$A_R = A_p/A_m = L_R^2$	$A_R = 1$	
		$(Vol)_R = (Vol)_p/(Vol)_m = L_R^3$	$Vol_R = 1$	
Kinematic		$V_R = V_p/V_m = L_R/T_R = L_p T_m / L_m T_p$	$V_R = 1$	
		$\alpha_R = \alpha_p/\alpha_m = V_R/T_R = L_R/T_R^2$	$T_R = T_p/T_m = 1$ $\alpha_R = 1$	
		$Q_R = Q_p/Q_m = A_R V_R = L_R^3 / T_R$	$Q_R = 1$	
Dynamic	Pressure	$\rho_R V_R^2 / p_R = 1$; $p_R = \rho_R V_R^2$; $p_R = \rho_R$	$p_R = \rho_p/\rho_m = 1.059/0.999 = 1.06$	1.06
	Gravity	$V_R^2 / g_R L_R = 1$; $V_R^2 = L_R$	$V_R^2 = 1$	-
	Viscosity	$\rho_R V_R L_R/\mu_R = 1$; $V_R = \mu_R/\rho_R L_R = \upsilon_R/L_R = \upsilon_R$	$\upsilon_R = 0.0323$	-
	Surf.Ten. Cap.Rise	$\rho_R V_R^2 L_R^2 / \sigma_R = 1$ $\sigma_R = \rho_R V_R^2 L_R^2$	$\sigma_R = \rho_p/\rho_m = 1.06$	1.06
	Elasticity	$\rho_R V_R^2 / E_R = 1$; $E = \rho_R V_R^2$	$E = \rho_R = p_R = \sigma_R$	1.06
		Water in model	Blood in Prototype	Ratios (p/m)
Mass density ρ		0.999 gm/cc	0.999x1.06=1.059	$\rho_r = 1.059/0.999 = 1.06$
Kinematic Viscosity ν		0.0068 stoke	0.0068x4.75=0.0323	$\nu_r = 0.0323/0.0068 = 4.75$

The adjusted Output ratios will be different if this model will be used for other prototypes rather than an adult male.

Exhibit 2

PROTOCOL

Unit	Data Measured from calibrated model	Data Computed	Data Corrected (A)
Lungs	**Pressure (mm Hg)** Min = Max = **Velocity (cm/sec)** Min = Max = - - - - - -	- - - - - **Flow (cm^3/sec)** Min = Max = **Elasticity (cm)** Min = Max =	
Upper Body	**Pressure (mm Hg)** Min = Max = **Velocity (cm/sec)** Min = Max = - - - - - -	- - - - - **Flow (cm^3/sec)** Min = Max = **Elasticity (cm)** Min = Max =	
Lower Body	**Pressure (mm Hg)** Min = Max = **Velocity (cm/sec)** Min = Max = - - - - - -	- - - - - **Flow (cm^3/sec)** Min = Max = **Elasticity (cm)** Min = Max =	
Response to fluid volume in the system	Min Volume (cm^3): Max Volume(cm^3): Min Storage (cm^3): Max Storage (cm^3):	- - - -	
Reaction time to change pumping regime (sec)	Min = Max = Average =	- - -	

Exhibit 3

Unit	Data from TAD/TAH testing (B)	Error (A-B)	Permissible Error	Difference
Lungs	**Pressure (mm Hg)** Min = Max = **Velocity (cm/sec)** Min = Max = **Flow (cm³/sec)** Min = Max = **Elasticity (cm)** Min = Max =			
Upper Body	**Pressure (mm Hg)** Min = Max = **Velocity (cm/sec)** Min = Max = **Flow (cm³/sec)** Min = Max = **Elasticity (cm)** Min = Max =			
Lower Body	**Pressure (mm Hg)** Min = Max = **Velocity (cm/sec)** Min = Max = Flow (cm³/sec) Min = Max = **Elasticity (cm)** Min = Max =			
Response to fluid volume in the system	Min Volume (cm³): Max Volume (cm³): Min Storage (cm³): Max Storage (cm³):			
Reaction time to change pumping regime (sec)	Min = Max = Average =			

Exhibit 4

PRESSURE IN HOMOLOGOUS POINTS Page 3 of 3

System	Point	Prototype	Model	Difference
Arteries	1			
	2			
	3			
	4			
	5			
	6			
	7			
	8			
	9			
	10			
	11			
Veins	12			
	13			
	14			
	15			
	16			
	17			
	18			
	19			
	20			
	21			
	22			

ANALYSIS OF RISKS

Statistics of Critical Point				Detectable Effect	Cumulative Effect	Risk		
Nr.	Parameter:					Low	Med	High
	Data	Avg.	St.Dev.					

Comments on Risks:

Statistics of Critical Point				Detectable Effect	Cumulative Effect	Risk		
Point	Parameter:					Low	Med	High
	Data	Avg.	St.Dev.					

Comments on Risks: _____

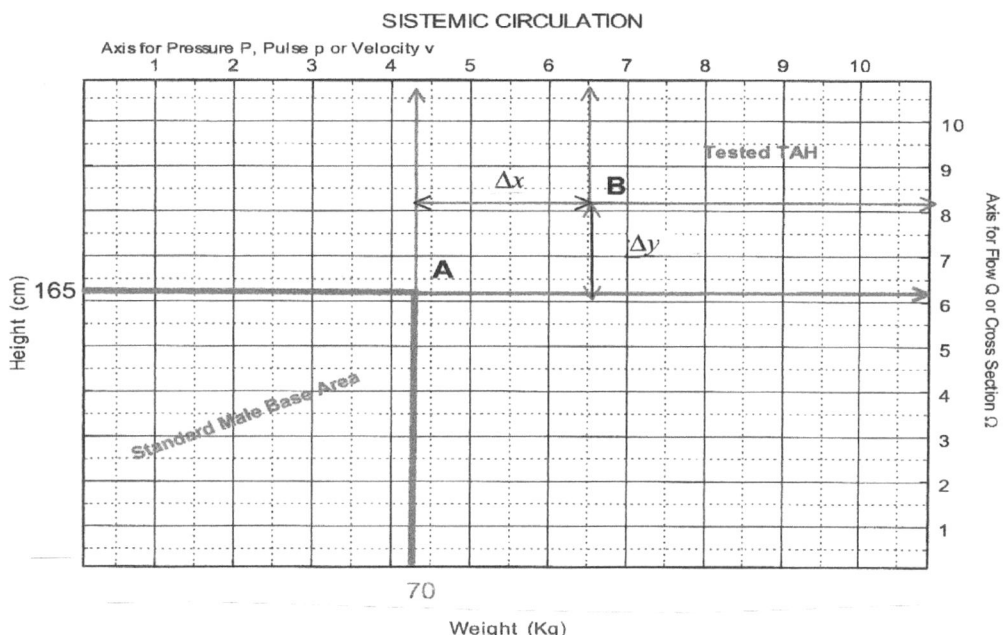

In the Exhibit 4 above 'difference' is Δx, and Δx Δy shows how the TAH differ from a normal individual we selected from Exhibit 5 and 6. Point B must coincide with A to have a match, if that does not happen the TAH must work better.

If we take the weight and height of a normal individual and plot versus some variables as those shown in the graph (P, p, v, Q and Ω) taken 22 homologous points Exhibit 4, the quantity of graphs as such will be 22 x 5 = 110.

Nonetheless, we can put a variable as function of another variable like v and Ω and reduce the quantity of graphs to 22 x 3 = 66. With four graphs of 4 axis we can reduce more yet. Plotting multiple curve lines per graph in each we will have less graphs for analysis. Many A's and B's may coincide then the graphs quantity even less, but this way of analysis could not work easily.

Because output data from testing a TAH is electronic, all this processing will be programed in such a way that graphs could be printed when needed and analysis will be made in the monitor.

Abnormal functioning of heart, sistemic and/or pulmonary circulation, to be identified and quantified by a funcioning Bench, to develop a prognosis and select a procedure for correction, is early to say at this time.

Exhibit 5

ULTRASOUND SCREENING FOR HEART AND VASCULAR SYSTEM									
Males									
Size / Number	Height m	Weight Kg	Pressure mm/Hg	Pulse per sec	Velocity cm/sec	Cross Section cm^2	Flow cm^3/s	OK Y / N	Obs
M30		30							
M40		40							
M50		50							
M60		60							
M70		70							
M80		80							
M90		90							
M100		100							
M110		110							
M120		120							
M130		130							
M135		135							
M140		140							
M145		145							
M150		150							
M155		155							
M160		160							

For each weight line, there are several heights not listed here.

MODEL POINT NUMBER:………………..

Exhibit 6

ULTRASOUND SCREENING FOR HEART AND VASCULAR SYSTEM									
Females									
Size / Number	Height m	Weight Kg	Pressure mm/Hg	Pulse per sec	Velocity cm/sec	Cross Section cm²	Flow cm³/s	OK Y / N	Obs.
F20		20							
F30		30							
F40		40							
F50		50							
F60		60							
F70		70							
F80		80							
F90		90							
F100		100							
F110		110							
F120		120							
F125		125							
F130		130							
F135		135							
F140		140							
F145		145							
F150		150							

For each weight line, there are several heights not listed here.

MODEL POINT NUMBER:………………..

ANNEX 2

Artificial heart – A History

From Wikipedia, the free encyclopedia

This article is about the mechanical device. For the Jonathan Coulton album, see Artificial Heart (album).

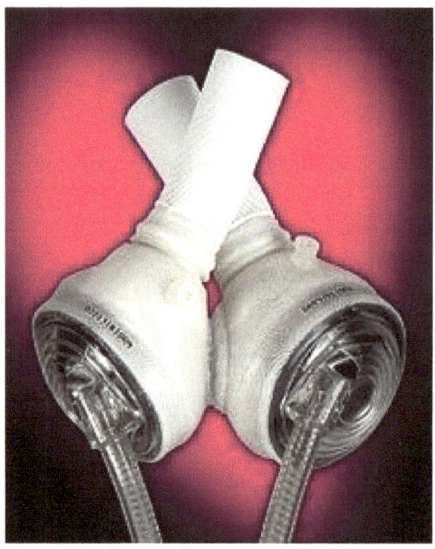

The SynCardia temporary Total Artificial Heart

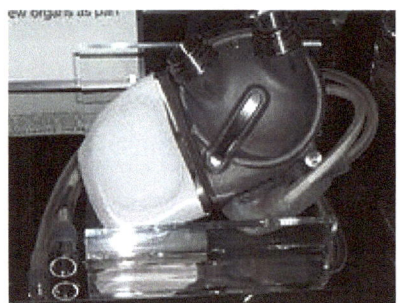

An artificial heart displayed at the London Science Museum

An **artificial heart** is a device that replaces the heart. Artificial hearts are typically used to bridge the time to heart transplantation, or to permanently replace the heart in case heart transplantation is impossible. Although other similar inventions preceded it going back to the late 1940s, the first artificial heart to be successfully implanted in a human was the Jarvik-7 in 1982, designed by a team including Willem Johan Kolff and Robert Jarvik.

An artificial heart is distinct from a ventricular assist device designed to support a failing heart. It is also distinct from a cardiopulmonary bypass machine, which is an external device used to provide the functions of both the heart and lungs and are used only for a few hours at a time, most commonly during cardiac surgery.

Contents

- 1 History
    - 1.1 Origins
    - 1.2 Early development
    - 1.3 Early designs of total artificial hearts
    - 1.4 First clinical implantation of a total artificial heart
    - 1.5 First clinical applications of a permanent pneumatic total artificial heart
    - 1.6 First clinical application of an intrathoracic pump
    - 1.7 First clinical application of a paracorporeal pump
    - 1.8 First VAD patient with FDA approved hospital discharge
- 2 Total artificial heart prototypes
    - 2.1 POLVAD
    - 2.2 Phoenix-7
    - 2.3 Abiomed AbioCor
    - 2.4 SynCardia
    - 2.5 MagScrew
    - 2.6 Abiomed AbioCor II
    - 2.7 Carmat bioprosthetic heart
    - 2.8 Frazier-Cohn
- 3 Others
    - 3.1 Hybrid assistive devices
- 4 See also
- 5 References
- 6 External links

History

Origins

A synthetic replacement for the heart remains one of the long-sought "holy grails" of modern medicine. The obvious benefit of a functional artificial heart would be to lower the need for heart transplants, because the demand for organs always greatly exceeds supply.

Although the heart is conceptually a pump, it embodies subtleties that defy straightforward emulation with synthetic materials and power supplies. Consequences of these issues include severe foreign-body rejection and external batteries that limit mobility. These complications limited the lifespan of early human recipients to hours or days.

Early development

The first artificial heart was made by the Soviet scientist Vladimir Demikhov in 1937. It was transplanted to a dog.

On July 3, 1952, 41-year-old Henry Opitek, suffering from shortness of breath, made medical history at Harper University Hospital at Wayne State University in Michigan. TheDodrill-GMR heart machine, considered to be the first operational mechanical heart, was successfully used while performing heart surgery.

Forest Dewey Dodrill, working closely with Matthew Dudley, used the machine in 1952 to bypass Henry Opitek's left ventricle for 50 minutes while he opened the patient's left atrium and worked to repair the mitral valve. In Dodrill's post-operative report, he notes, "To our knowledge, this is the first instance of survival of a patient when a mechanicaly heart mechanism was used to take over the complete body function of maintaining the blood supply of the body while the heart was open and operated on.

A heart–lung machine was first used in 1953 during a successful open heart surgery. John Heysham Gibbon, the inventor of the machine, performed the operation and developed the heart–lung substitute himself.

Following these advances, scientific interest for the development of a solution for heart disease developed in numerous research groups worldwide.

Early designs of total artificial hearts

In 1949, a precursor to the modern artificial heart pump was built by doctors William Sewell and William Glenn of the Yale School of Medicine using an Erector Set, assorted odds and ends, and dime-store toys. The external pump successfully bypassed the heart of a dog for more than an hou.

Paul Winchell invented an artificial heart with the assistance of Henry Heimlich (the inventor of the Heimlich Maneuver) and held the first patent for such a device. The University of Utah developed a similar apparatus around the same time, but when they tried to patent it, Winchell's heart was cited as prior art. The university requested that Winchell donate the heart to the University of Utah, which he did. There is some debate as to how much of Winchell's design Robert Jarvik used in creating Jarvik's artificial heart. Heimlich states, "I saw the heart, I saw the patent and I saw the letters. The basic principle used in Winchell's heart and Jarvik's heart is exactly the same. Jarvik denies that any of Winchell's design elements were incorporated into the device he fabricated for humans which was successfully implanted into Barney Clark in 1982.

On December 12, 1957, Willem Johan Kolff, the world's most prolific inventor of artificial organs, implanted an artificial heart into a dog at Cleveland Clinic. The dog lived for 90 minutes.

In 1958, Domingo Liotta initiated the studies of TAH replacement at Lyon, France, and in 1959–60 at the National University of Córdoba, Argentina. He presented his work at the meeting of the American Society for Artificial Internal Organs held in Atlantic City in March 1961. At that meeting, Liotta described the implantation of three types of orthotopic (inside the pericardial sac) TAHs in dogs, each of which used a different source of external energy: an implantable electric motor, an implantable rotating pump with an external electric motor, and a pneumatic pump.

In 1964, the National Institutes of Health started the Artificial Heart Program, with the goal of putting a man-made heart into a human by the end of the decade. The purpose of the program was to develop an implantable artificial heart, including the power source, to replace a failing heart.

In February 1966, Adrian Kantrowitz rose to international prominence when he performed the world's first permanent implantation of a partial mechanical heart (left ventricular assist device) at Maimonides Medical Center.

In 1967, Kolff left Cleveland Clinic to start the Division of Artificial Organs at the University of Utah and pursue his work on the artificial heart.

1. In 1973, a calf named Tony survived for 30 days on an early Kolff heart.
2. In 1975, a bull named Burk survived 90 days on the artificial heart.
3. In 1976, a calf named Abebe lived for 184 days on the Jarvik 5 artificial heart.
4. In 1981, a calf named Alfred Lord Tennyson lived for 268 days on the Jarvik 5.

Over the years, more than 200 physicians, engineers, students and faculty developed, tested and improved Kolff's artificial heart. To help manage his many endeavors, Kolff assigned project managers. Each project was named after its manager. Graduate student Robert Jarvik was the project manager for the artificial heart, which was subsequently renamed the Jarvik 7.

In 1981, William DeVries submitted a request to the FDA for permission to implant the Jarvik 7 into a human being. On December 2, 1982, Kolff implanted the Jarvik 7 artificial heart into Barney Clark, a dentist from Seattle who was suffering from severe congestive heart failure. Clark lived for 112 days tethered to an external pneumatic compressor, a device weighing some 400 pounds (180 kg), but during that time he suffered prolonged periods of confusion and a number of instances of bleeding, and asked several times to be allowed to die.

First clinical implantation of a total artificial heart

On April 4, 1969, Domingo Liotta and Denton A. Cooley replaced a dying man's heart with a mechanical heart inside the chest at The Texas Heart Institute in Houston as a bridge for a transplant. The man woke up and began to recover. After 64 hours, the pneumatic-powered artificial heart was removed and replaced by a donor heart. However thirty-two hours after transplantation, the man died of what was later proved to be an acute pulmonary infection, extended to both lungs, caused by fungi, most likely caused by an immunosuppressive drug complication.

The original prototype of Liotta-Cooley artificial heart used in this historic operation is prominently displayed in the Smithsonian Institution's National Museum of American History "Treasures of American History" exhibit in Washington, D.C.

First clinical applications of a permanent pneumatic total artificial heart

The first clinical use of an artificial heart designed for permanent implantation rather than a bridge to transplant occurred in 1982 at the University of Utah. Artificial kidney pioneer Willem Johan Kolff started the Utah artificial organs program in 1967. There, physician-engineer Clifford Kwan-Gett invented two components of an integrated pneumatic artificial heart system: a ventricle with hemispherical diaphragms that did not crush red blood cells (a problem with previous artificial hearts) and an external heart driver that inherently regulated blood flow without needing complex control systems. Independently, Paul Winchell designed and patented a similarly shaped ventricle and donated the patent to the Utah program. Throughout the 1970s and early 1980s, veterinarian Donald Olsen led a series of calf experiments that refined the artificial heart and its surgical care. During that time, as a student at the University of Utah, Robert Jarvik combined several modifications: an ovoid shape to fit inside the human chest, a more blood-compatible polyurethane developed by biomedical engineer Donald Lyman, and a fabrication method by Kwan-Gett that made the inside of the ventricles smooth and seamless to reduce dangerous stroke-causing blood clots. On December 2, 1982, William DeVries implanted the artificial heart into retired dentist Barney Bailey Clark (born January 21, 1921), who survived 112 days with the device, dying on March 23, 1983. Bill Schroeder became the second recipient and lived for a record 620 days.

Contrary to popular belief and erroneous articles in several periodicals, the Jarvik heart was not banned for permanent use. Today, the modern version of the Jarvik 7 is known as the SynCardia temporary Total Artificial Heart. It has been implanted in more than 1,350 people as a bridge to transplantation.

In the mid-1980s, artificial hearts were powered by dishwasher-sized pneumatic power sources whose lineage went back to Alfa Laval milking machines. Moreover, two sizable catheters had to cross the body wall to carry the pneumatic pulses to the implanted heart, greatly increasing the risk of infection. To speed development of a new generation of technologies, the National Heart, Lung, and Blood Institute opened a competition for implantable electrically powered artificial hearts. Three groups received funding: Cleveland Clinic in Cleveland, Ohio; the College of Medicine of Pennsylvania State University (Penn State Hershey Medical Center) in Hershey, Pennsylvania; and AbioMed, Inc. of Danvers, Massachusetts. Despite considerable progress, the Cleveland program was discontinued after the first five years.

Polymeric trileaflet valves ensure unidirectional blood flow with a low pressure gradient and good longevity. State-of-the-art transcutaneous energy transfer eliminates the need for electric wires crossing the chest wall.

First clinical application of an intrathoracic pump

On July 19, 1963, E. Stanley Crawford and Domingo Liotta implanted the first clinical Left Ventricular Assist Device (LVAD) at The Methodist Hospital in Houston, Texas, in a patient who had a cardiac arrest after surgery. The patient survived for four days under mechanical support but did not recover from the complications of the cardiac arrest; finally, the pump was discontinued, and the patient died.

First clinical application of a paracorporeal pump

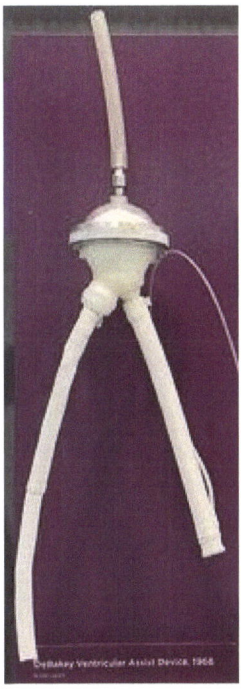

1966 DeBakey ventricular assist device

On April 21, 1966, Michael DeBakey and Liotta implanted the first clinical LVAD in a paracorporeal position (where the external pump rests at the side of the patient) at The Methodist Hospital in Houston, in a patient experiencing cardiogenic shock after heart surgery. The patient developed neurological and pulmonary complications and died after few days of LVAD mechanical support. In October 1966, DeBakey and Liotta implanted the paracorporeal Liotta-DeBakey LVAD in a new patient who recovered well and was discharged from the hospital after 10 days of mechanical support, thus constituting the first successful use of an LVAD for postcardiotomy shock.

First VAD patient with FDA approved hospital discharge

In 1990 Brian Williams was discharged from the University of Pittsburgh Medical Center (UPMC), becoming the first VAD patient to be discharged with Food and Drug Administration (FDA) approval. The patient was supported in part by bioengineers from the University of Pittsburgh's McGowan Institute.

Total artificial heart prototypes

POLVAD

Since 1991, the Foundation for Cardiac Surgery Development (FRK) in Zabrze, Poland has been working on developing an artificial heart. Nowadays, the Polish system for heart support POLCAS consists of the artificial ventricle POLVAD-MEV and the three controllers POLPDU-401, POLPDU-402 and POLPDU-501. Presented devices are designed to handle only one patient. The control units of the 401 and 402 series may be used only in hospital due to its big size, method of control and type of power supply. The control unit of 501 series is the latest product of FRK. Due to its much smaller size and weight, it is significantly more mobile solution. For this reason, it can be also used during supervised treatment conducted outside the hospital.

Phoenix-7

In June 1996, a 46-year-old man received a total artificial heart implantation done by Jeng Wei at Cheng-Hsin General Hospital in the Republic of China (Taiwan). This technologically advanced pneumatic Phoenix-7 Total Artificial Heart was manufactured by a Taiwanese dentist Kelvin K. Cheng, a Chinese physician T. M. Kao and colleagues at the Taiwan TAH Research Center in Tainan, Republic of China (Taiwan). With this experimental artificial heart, the patient's BP was maintained at 90-100/40-55 mmHg and cardiac output at 4.2–5.8 L/min. The patient then received the world's first successful combined heart and kidney transplantation after bridging with a total artificial heart.

Abiomed AbioCor

The first AbioCor to be surgically implanted in a patient was on July 3, 2001. [25] The AbioCor is made of titanium and plastic with a weight of two pounds, and its internal battery can be recharged with a transduction device that sends power through the skin.[1] The internal battery lasts for a half-hour, and a wearable external battery pack lasts for four hours. The FDA announced on September 5, 2006, that the AbioCor could be implanted for humanitarian uses after the device had been tested on 15 patients. It is intended for critically ill patients who cannot receive a heart transplant. Some limitations of the current AbioCor are that its size makes it suitable for only about 50% of the male population, and its useful life is only 1–2 years.

SynCardia

SynCardia is a company based in Tucson, Arizona which currently has two separate models available. It is available in a 70cc and 50cc size. The 70 cc is used for biventricular heart failure in adult men, while the 50cc is for children and women. As good results with the TAH as a bridge to heart transplant accumulated, a trial of the CardioWest TAH (developed from the Jarvik 7 and now marketed as the Syncardia TAH) was initiated in 1993 and completed in 2002. As of 2014, more than 1,250 patients have received SynCardia artificial hearts. The device requires the use of the Companion 2 hospital driver or the Freedom portable driver to power the heart with pulses of air. The drivers also monitor blood flow for each ventricle.

MagScrew

Another U.S. team has a prototype called the 2005 MagScrew Total Artificial Heart. Teams in Japan and South Korea are also racing to produce similar devices.

Abiomed AbioCor I

By combining its valved ventricles with the control technology and roller screw developed at Penn State, AbioMed has designed a smaller, more stable heart, the AbioCor II. This pump, which should be implantable in most men and 50% of women with a life span of up to five years, had animal trials in 2005, and the company hoped to get FDA approval for human use in 2008.

Carmat bioprosthetic heart

On October 27, 2008, French professor and leading heart transplant specialist Alain F. Carpentier announced that a fully implantable artificial heart would be ready for clinical trial by 2011 and for alternative transplant in 2013. It was developed and would be manufactured by him, biomedical firm CARMAT SA, and venture capital firm Truffle Capital. The prototype used embedded electronic sensors and was made from chemically treated animal tissues, called "biomaterials", or a "pseudo-skin" of biosynthetic, microporous materials.

According to a press-release by Carmat dated December 20, 2013, the first implantation of its artificial heart in a 75-year-old patient was performed on December 18, 2013 by the Georges Pompidou European Hospital team in Paris (France). The patient died 75 days after the operation.

In Carmat's design, two chambers are each divided by a membrane that holds hydraulic fluid on one side. A motorized pump moves hydraulic fluid in and out of the chambers, and that fluid causes the membrane to move; blood flows through the other side of each membrane. The blood-facing side of the membrane is made of tissue obtained from a sac that surrounds a cow's heart, to make the device more biocompatible. The Carmat device also uses valves made from cow heart tissue and has sensors to detect increased pressure within the device. That information is sent to an internal control system that can adjust the flow rate in response to increased demand, such as when a patient is exercising. This distinguishes it from previous designs that maintain a constant flow rate.

The Carmat device, unlike previous designs, is meant to be used in cases of terminal heart failure, instead of being used as a bridge device while the patient awaits a transplant. At 900 grams it weighs nearly three times the typical heart and is targeted primarily towards obese men. It also requires the patient to carry around an additional Li-Ion battery. The projected lifetime of the artificial heart is around 5 years (230 million beats).

Frazier-Cohn]

On 12 March 2011, an experimental artificial heart was implanted in 55-year-old Craig Lewis at The Texas Heart Institute in Houston by Drs. O. H. Frazier and William Cohn. The device is a combination of two modified HeartMate II pumps that is currently undergoing bovine trials.

Frazier and Cohn are on the board of the BiVACOR company that develops an artificial heart. BiVACOR has been tested as a replacement for a heart in a sheep. So far, only one person has benefited from Frazier and Cohn's artificial heart. Craig Lewis was suffering from amyloidosis in 2011 when his heart gave out and doctors pronounced that he had only 12 to 24 hours to live. After obtaining permission from his family, Frazier and Cohn replaced his heart with their device. Lewis survived for another 5 weeks after the operation; he eventually succumbed to liver and kidney failure due to his amyloidosis, after which his family asked that his artificial heart be unplugged.

Others

A centrifugal pump or an axial-flow pump can be used as an artificial heart, resulting in the patient being alive without a pulse.

A centrifugal artificial heart which alternately pumps the pulmonary circulation and the systemic circulation, causing a pulse has been described. Researchers have constructed a heart out of foam. The heart is made out of flexible silicone and works with an external pump to push air and fluids through the heart. It currently cannot be implanted into humans, but it is a promising start for artificial hearts.

Hybrid assistive devices

Patients who have some remaining heart function but who can no longer live normally may be candidates for ventricular assist devices (VAD), which do not replace the human heart but complement it by taking up much of the function.

The first Left Ventricular Assist Device (LVAD) system was created by Domingo Liotta at Baylor College of Medicine in Houston in 1962Another VAD, the Kantrowitz CardioVad, designed by Adrian Kantrowitz boosts the native heart by taking up over 50% of its function. Additionally, the VAD can help patients on the wait list for a heart transplant. In a young person, this device could delay the need for a transplant by 10–15 years, or even allow the heart to recover, in which case the VAD can be removed. The artificial heart is powered by a battery that needs to be changed several times while still working.

The first heart assist device was approved by the FDA in 1994, and two more received approval in 1998. While the original assist devices emulated the pulsating heart, newer versions, such as the Heartmate II, developed by The Texas Heart Institute of Houston, provide continuous flow. These pumps (which may be centrifugal or axial flow) are smaller and potentially more durable and last longer than the current generation of total heart replacement pumps. Another major advantage of a VAD is that the patient keeps the natural heart, which may still function for temporary back-up support if the mechanical pump were to stop. This may provide enough support to keep the patient alive until a solution to the problem is implemented.

In August 2006, an artificial heart was implanted into a 15-year-old girl at the Stollery Children's Hospital in Edmonton, Alberta. It was intended to act as a temporary fixture until a donor heart could be found. Instead, the artificial heart (called a Berlin Heart) allowed for natural processes to occur and her heart healed on its own. After 146 days, the Berlin Heart was removed, and the girl's heart was able to function properly on its own. [1]On December 16, 2011 the Berlin Heart gained U.S. FDA approval. The device has since been successfully implanted in several children including a 4-year-old Honduran girl at Children's Hospital Boston.

Several continuous-flow ventricular assist devices have been approved for use in the European Union, and, as of August 2007, were undergoing clinical trials for FDA approval.

In 2012, a study published in the New England Journal of Medicine compared the Berlin Heart to extracorporeal membrane oxygenation (ECMO) and concluded that "a ventricular assist device available in several sizes for use in children as a bridge to heart transplantation [such as the Berlin Heart] was associated with a significantly higher rate of survival as compared with ECMO." The study's primary author, Charles D. Fraser, Jr., surgeon in chief at Texas Children's Hospital, explained: "With the Berlin Heart, we have a more effective therapy to offer patients earlier in the management of their heart failure. When we sit with parents, we have real data to offer so they can make an informed decision. This is a giant step forward."

Suffering from end-stage heart failure, former Vice President Dick Cheney underwent a procedure in July 2010 to have a VAD implanted at INOVA Fairfax Hospital, in Fairfax Virginia. In 2012, he received a heart transplant at age 71 after 20 months on a waiting list.

Annex 3

REFERENCES

THE UNIVERSITY OF UTAH

INSTITUTE FOR BIOMEDICAL ENGINEERING
(AN INTERCOLLEGE INSTITUTE) AND
DIVISION OF ARTIFICIAL ORGANS
DEPARTMENT OF SURGERY

WILLEM J. KOLFF, M.D., PH.D.
DISTINGUISHED PROFESSOR AND DIRECTOR
DUMKE BUILDING 535
1920 E. NORTH CAMPUS DRIVE
SALT LAKE CITY, UT 84112
PHONE: (801) 581-6296

June 23, 1981

To Whom it May Concern:

This is an official invitation to Professor Samuel Gueller to come to the Institute for Biomedical Engineering and the Division of Artificial Organs of the University of Utah, Salt Lake City, Utah, U.S.A. I have been very impressed by the design of a novel blood pump that Dr. Samuel Gueller has sent me. Indeed, since this is such a novel pump, the consequences of its further investigation might be very important for the field of artificial organs in general and the artificial heart in particular.

Sincerely yours,

WILLEM J. KOLFF, M.D., Ph.D.

WJK:jh

Presentation letter by Dr. Willem J. Kolff

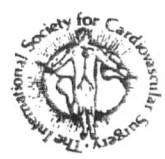 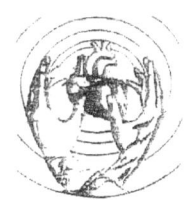 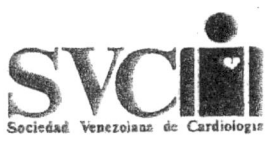

INTERNATIONAL SOCIETY FOR CARDIOVASCULAR SURGERY
XVII CONGRESO DEL CAPITULO LATINOAMERICANO

SOCIEDAD VENEZOLANA DE CARDIOLOGIA
XIII JORNADAS NACIONALES

SOCIEDAD VENEZOLANA DE ANGIOLOGIA Y CIRUGIA CARDIOVASCULAR
II CONGRESO

Caracas, Septiembre 30 – Octubre 4– 1.984

CONSTANCIA

Que se expide a:

DR. SAMUEL GUELLER

Por su asistencia y participación en estos eventos, celebrados en la ciudad de Caracas, del 30 de septiembre al 4 de octubre de 1984.

P/Comité Organizador

Dr. Ruben Jaén Centeno
Presidente
XVII CONGRESO LATINOAMERICANO

Dr. Domingo Navarro Dona
Presidente
XIII JORNADAS DE CARDIOLOGIA

Congress Paper on an Electric Powered, Non-Transcutaneous wiring TAH

SERIAL NUMBER	FILING DATE	GRP ART UNIT	FIL FEE REC'D	ATTORNEY DOCKET NO.	DRWGS	TOT CL	IND CL
06/497,512	05/24/83	336	$ 300.00	529 EAG	9	12	1

ERNEST A. GREENSIDE
19 WEST 34TH ST.
NEW YORK, NY 10001

RECEIVED
JUN 22 1983
ERNEST A. GREENSIDE

Receipt is acknowledged of the patent application identified herein. It will be considered in its order and you will be notified as to the examination thereof. Be sure to give the U.S. SERIAL NUMBER, DATE OF FILING, NAME OF APPLICANT, and TITLE OF INVENTION when inquiring about this application. Fees transmitted by check or draft are subject to collection. Please verify the accuracy of the data presented on this transmittal.

Applicant(s)   SAMUEL GUELLER, CARACAS, VENEZUELA.

TITLE
COMPUTERIZED ARTIFICIAL HEART

Application for a Patent of a Computerized Artificial Heart with description of transcutaneous transfer of energy and use of a single miniature pump to operate the diaphragms with not role for air, as well as implantable hardware controls and programable software.

Notations

H, h = head

v = specific discharge

f = friction factor

D = diameter

d = discharge

g = acceleration of gravity

c = celerity

V, v, υ = velocity

T = time

κ = intrinsic permeability

υ = kinematic viscosity

φ = head in matrix media

P, p = pressure

z = height from reference level

E = elasticity coefficient

S = drawdown, suction

k = coefficient of permeability

d = thickness of layer

Q = flow per unit time

r = radius of the vessel

L = length

η = viscosity

ΔxΔy = area increment

BIBLIOGRAPHY

ASCE Manual of Engineering Practice Nr. 97. Hydraulic Modeling Concepts and Practice, 2000

Burton, A. C., Physiology and Biophysics of the Circulation, Year Book Medical Publishers, Chicago, 1972

Campbell, F. B. and Pickett, E. B. Prototype Performance and Model-Prototype Relationship. McGraw-Hill, New York, 1969

Halliwell, A.R., Velocity of a Water-Hammer Wave in an Elastic Pipe, Journal of the Hydraulics Division, ASCE, pp. 1021, July 1963

Karplus, W. J., Analog Simulation, McGraw-Hill, New York, 1958

Kellog, O. D., Foundations of Potential Theory, Springer, 1929

Kenlegan, G. H., Wave Motion, John Wiley, New York, 1950

Langhaar, H.L., Dimensional Analysis and Theory of Models, John Wiley, New York, 1951

Maxwell, W. H. C. and Weggel, J. R., Surface Tension in Froude Models, Journal of the Hydraulics Division, ASCE, pp. 677-701, March 1969

Paynter, Henry M., Fluid Transients in Engineering Systems, McGraw-Hill, New York, 1961

Raghunath, H. M., Dimensional Analysis and Hydraulic Model Testing, Asia Publishing House, New York, 1967

Southwell, R.V., Relaxation Methods in Engineering Science, Oxford University Press, 1940

Vogel, Steven, Vital Circuits, Oxford University Press, 1992

Waite L. and Fine J., Applied Biofluids Mechanics, McGraw-Hill, New York, 2007

William, Vallee L., Expert Panel Review of the NHLBI Total Artificial Heart (TAH) Program, National Institute of Health, November 1999

Wood, Don J., Dorsch, R. G., and Lightner, Charlene, Wave-Plan Analysis of Unsteady Flow in Closed Conduits, Journal of the Hydraulics Division, ASCE, pp. 83-110, March 1966

About the Author

Sam Gueller was born in Argentina where he studied Land Surveying and Civil Engineering, later he continues studies at the University of Cincinnati, University of California, University of Delft (Holland), Technion University (Israel) and University of Graz (Austria). He has twelve years' experience as Assistant Professor, worked for Consulting firms, and has been staff International Specialist in the Inter-American Development Bank.

Fellowships: Government of Argentina, Government of The Netherlands, Government of Israel, Government of Austria, State of Ohio, President of the University of Cincinnati. He has working experience in fifteen countries and four States in the U.S., and have interest in science and technology. He made math and analog modeling of several phenomena particularly in Fluid Mechanics and authored books and papers in many Congresses, domestic and abroad. He is a Life Member of the American Society of Civil Engineers, Member of the Asociación Física Argentina, and other professional societies.

Dr. Gueller and wife reside part time in USA and Argentina.

www.ingramcontent.com/pod-product-compliance
Lightning Source LLC
Chambersburg PA
CBHW051202220526
45473CB00003B/866